KETO FOR CANCER

Metabolic ketogenic diet against cancer cells to live in health

Enric Scott

CONTENTS
Introduction

Chapter 1 -
What is cancer?
How cancer cells travel? Metastasis
Do you know about Cancer metabolism?
Mitochondrial metabolic disturbances: one of the causes of cancer
Defective uncontrolled inflammatory response as one of the causes of cancer
The 10 terrain of cancer

Chapter 2 -
Is glucose the reason for proliferation of Cancer cell? The science behind Keto diet
How does cancer cells are flourish with the help of glucose and glutamine?
Another fuel driving cancer: glutamine
What goes wrong with glucose metabolism?

Chapter 3 -
What causes Cancer?
How is a tumor formed?
Can we prevent cancer?

Chapter 4 -
Is ketosis a way of fasting to starve cancer cells?
Benefits of fasting
Few things to know before fasting
Types of fasting
Which is the most adaptable way of fasting?

Chapter 5 -
What is ketogenic diet?
Process of ketosis
What is the reason behind consuming lot of fats?
Why should you take protein in a moderate quantity?
Is ketogenic diet helpful- only in weight loss?

Chapter 6 -
What is important for keto diet?
Medical fitness
Right food
Right plans

Chapter 7 -
How does ketogenic diet work against cancer?
Are you starting a ketogenic diet to prevent cancer?
Know this:
Testing for ketosis

Chapter 8 -
Is keto diet always beneficial?
Benefits of keto diet
Side effects of keto diet
Is ketogenic diet dangerous? Find out that it is a myth or truth.
Ketoacidosis (its effect)

Chapter 9 -
How does ketogenic diet works for losing weight?
What should you do if you stop losing weight on a keto diet?

Chapter 10 -
Do you want to live a cancer free life? Follow the tips.
How long should you remain on ketogenic diet?
Long term rewards of ketogenic diet

Conclusion

Keto Recipes

INTRODUCTION

Since ancient times, fasting was practiced for curing many ailments. A fat high and low carbohydrate diet is assumed to be an alternative of fasting or starvation, having many of the same desired effect simultaneously nourishing the cells. One of the most dangerous nutritional myths is that our body needs a continuous supply of carbohydrate and glucose. Therefore, we make carbohydrate as our staple diet making it as 45 to 65% of our total calorie. This is false!

Ketogenic metabolic therapy has been introduced that is proposed by a group of clinical who wants to emphasize the use of ketogenic nutritional intervention as an anticancer therapy. This new strategy exploits cancer metabolic cravings for glucose and other fuels that can ferment. A contradiction to this therapy, 'American cancer society', recommends that individuals with cancer can eat whatever they want! Like really? If you also think so then there is no use of reading this book. But if, you have trust in me then keep reading for more guidance of how to adapt ketogenic diet for anticancer life? The term ketogenic diet was later coined by Wilder and Peterman. The formulated the fat to carbohydrate ratios i.e., 1 g protein per kg of body weight in children and 10 to 15 gram carbohydrates daily and fat should be for the remainder of calories. This ratio is still used today and has reportedly approved the improvement in patient's mental activity and cognition.

Nothing wants to work hard, right? Your system is quite capable of converting fats into energy but, it is harder than converting glucose for energy. Fat metabolism required an adequate amount of raw material; therefore, your body is dependent on glucose. At first, when you are deprived of carbohydrates your body will fight back and cause some side effects. It slowly starts to adjust to the new metabolism of burning fat, whether, it is dietary or body fat and this process is called **ketosis.**

There are certain fundamentals which you should know about the food you eat. You must have heard about macro nutrients and micro nutrients. Macro nutrients are those elements which are present in a large amount of the food (carbohydrates, protein and fat), and micro nutrients are those elements which are present and needed in a very low quantity (vitamins and minerals). We need large amount of macronutrients, as it provides fuel to our body to produce energy. Our body finds it very easy to burn glucose for producing energy. It sounds simple and natural but since man has become more and more dependent on glucose we have seen a dramatic rise in the incident of diabetes heart disease and obesity. Nowadays many doctors and society scientists are beginning to believe that all the diseases are linked with excess of carbohydrate consumption, and that a ketogenic diet is both the answer and cure. They have formulated certain rules in this diet to put stress on diseased cells to stop their growth.

CHAPTER 1

What is cancer?

According to American cancer society it is a collection of over hundred different diseases and imbalances in your body. But, according to most recent research it is demonstrated that cancel is rather a singular disease of energy metabolism. All types of cancer May it was in tissue or cellular level use fermentation (the Warburg effect) to produce energy which is different from how our body cells generally produce energy. Cancer is broadly defined as uncontrolled division of abnormal cells which spread throughout the body forming a mass of cells called a tumor. This tumor, when grow and expand, can affect the surrounding normal tissues or organs such as liver or bowel.

There are over 200 known type of cancers, and specific traits have been identified with which they are inherent to each one. These are called Hallmark of Cancer cells which a cell must possess in order to become cancerous. Healthy cells have 10 different security systems in place to keep cancer from taking over there function. This is why we all don't have a full-blown diagnosable cancer despite the aforementioned presence of cancer cells in our body. In 2000 Douglas Hanahan and Robert Weinberg published a ground-breaking review article in the journal cell in which they are identified the original 6 Hallmarks of cancerous cell. In 2011, they were, updated their list by proposing to four more.

The main characteristics/hallmarks of cancer/cancerous cells are -

- Cancer cells control their own rate of proliferation

(they multiply without creating protein that encourages their explosive growth)

- They have the ability to escape from cell apoptosis - normal cells kill themselves when they detect error like mutation which cannot be repaired but cancer cells do not kill themselves, even though they have mutation rather they collect mutation and gain benefit from them to thrive on any condition.

- Do not respond to cell inhibitory signal - they disarm the process that our body uses to put a break on unwanted cell division.

- Have unlimited replication potential - normal cells die after a certain number of divisions but this characteristic is absent in cancer cells, and they are immortal.

- Can spread and travel from the site of origin (known as metastasize) - this spread in the sites were space, oxygen and nutrition are available in a plenty amount.

- Promote the process of angiogenesis - when tumor grows it blocks the supply of blood vessels so it grows new blood vessels needed to sustain them.

- Re programs energy metabolism (known as Warburg effect) - these cells change their method of energy production and increase their metabolic rate in order to sustain themselves.

- Evading from immune destruction - cancer cells suppress the function of immune cells, including natural killer cells and escapes from immune surveillance system which results in weakening of immune system.

- Mutation of genome - these cells have defected capability to repair DNA allowing the reproduction of mutated cells.

- Inflammation of area around tumor- tumor activates an inflammatory response that can increase their access to growth factors and blood supply.

In general these 10 hallmarks of Cancer are largely accepted by Western medicine. Our aim is little different from Western medicines as they are a drug approach to cancer but in this book we will have a nutritional approach to prevent cancer!

Cancer commonly can take some months, sometime years to develop into a mass which can be diagnosed. A person who looks healthy can even produce 500-1000 new cancerous cell per day! And only 1000 people truly are cancer free. It is shocking to know that we all have cancer cells in our body no matter how healthy we are. All cancer cells require a kick to proliferate to turn into an uncontrollable growing mass of cells. In this book we will learn how to control our self to save us from cancer.

How Cancer Cells Travel? Metastasis:

Blood vessels serve as the body's highway system. Blood pumped from the heart is carried to distant tissues and organs by a vast network of blood vessels that includes nineteen billion capillaries. When a tumor metastasizes, and enters either the blood vessel superhighway or the lymphatic system to travel to a new location. This is how they form new tumors in different parts of the body. For example, if liver cancer spreads to the breasts, it is called metastatic liver cancer, not breast cancer.

Like explorers hungry to discover new lands, a growing tumor will designate clusters of pioneer cells to travel to distant body parts where they can form new tumor, or secondary tumors. It's how the West was won—not a new concept. But how do cancer cells go about it? Remember that a large proportion of human tissue has extracellular space filled with carbohydrate and protein molecules called the ECM. Molecules in ECM tether themselves to one another, forming thick web like bonds. In order for cancer cells to metastasize, they must break these bonds by creating protein-digesting enzymes. Like swordsmen through the jungle, cancer cells hack away at the thick matrix. Once they've escaped from the matrix, metastatic cancer cells attempt to gain access to systemic circulation by one of two routes. For many cancer cells, their best opportunity to spread is by means of the lymphatic system (this is why lymph nodes are often biopsied or removed during the surgery to assess if the cancer has spread; this information also determines the cancer's stage). Using the alternative route, cancer cells enter the bloodstream either indirectly through the lymph or directly through blood vessels.

Once these pioneer cancer cells arrive at a distant organ, they can grow into a metastatic tumor. But most of them do not. It has been estimated that between ten million and one billion cancer cells are released into the bloodstream by tumors on a daily basis, but only 0.001 percent go on to develop into metastatic colonies. A century ago Dr. Stephen Paget, a surgeon, asserted the "seed and soil" hypothesis. He theorized that the organ preference patterns of metastasizing tumors are due to symbiotic interactions between the metastatic tumor cell (the seed) and its potential new organ micro environment (the soil). Some tumor types are able to form metastases in just about any organ in the body, but the most frequently targeted organs for the metastasis are bone, brain, liver, and lung. When a person's terrain is balanced and healthy, cancer can't form a metastatic tumor, as the new environment will not support it. Metastatic cancer cells are essentially seeds that grow into highly toxic, lethal plants only if they are planted in unhealthy soil.

A portion of the "soil", Dr. Paget referred it now as the tumor micro environment, or TME. The TME consists of all the noncancerous cells present within the tumor. These include immune cells, cytokines, growth factors, ROS, and other inflammatory compounds. One other compound found in the TME is the cancer-associated fibroblast (CAF). These are cells that promote the cancer process by encouraging tumor growth, angiogenesis, inflammation, and metastasis. Since they are associated with cancer at all stages of progression—their production of growth factors facilitates angiogenesis—they have become an emerging target for cancer therapies. In fact, normal fibroblasts (cells found in connective tissue that produce the collagen and fibers that make up the ECM) can be "educated" by cancer cells to express pro-inflammatory genes, further fuelling the cancer process.

There is a lot happening in the immediate surroundings, the soil, of a tumor that can help to either provoke or inhibits its growth. The metastatic cancer is favoured by an inflammated, immune-compromised, and highly oxidative surrounding. When the terrain is optimized, metastatic cancer cannot sprout. Because blood and the circulatory system are the primary systems that can enable cancer's growth and spread, understanding how blood flow works?—and how nutrition factors into it—is paramount.

DO YOU KNOW ABOUT CANCER METABOLISM?

Cancer is a disease in which cells lose their ability of controllable growth and divide continuously to form a mass of cell called tumor. Tumor is a mass of abnormal mutated cells which exhibit prolific growth. It is considered to be as a genetic disease which involves mutations in the nucleus of tumor suppressing genes and oncogenes, but experiments according to Otto Warburg proves that cancer is caused by mitochondria metabolic dysfunctioning.

MITOCHONDRIAL METABOLIC DISTURBANCES: ONE OF THE CAUSES OF CANCER

Otto Warburg was a German biochemistry who had special interest in the metabolism of Cancer cells he observed that cancer cells increase their rate of glucose fermentation even in the presence of a lot of oxygen verbals. This theory was based on his findings that cancer cells cannot use oxygen to produce energy via mitochondrial respiration. They rely on fermentation to obtain their energy in order to compensate their defective mitochondrial respiration. The dependence of cancerous cell on fermented products even in the presence of oxygen was referred to as Warburg effect.

Fermentation is the primitive process of respiration of glucose to obtain energy in the absence of oxygen but in humans fermentation by itself usually has a very low amount of energy yield. The increasing amount of dependence of cells on the fermented product indicated Warburg that there was something wrong with the energy house of the cell that is mitochondria. The switch of dependence on energy from mitochondrial ATP to fermented products indicates that something is wrong with the cell functions, and if a cell survives, it multiplies into a group of dysfunctional cells which can escape from cell apoptosis results in forming malignant tumor.

A growing tumor, starts blocking the blood containing oxygen and other vital nutrients and adapt themselves to thrive in a low oxygen environment. These cells then reprogram their cell metabolism and start surviving by developing new blood vessels network (called angiogenesis) to feed the lactic acid produced from the fermentation of glucose is toxic and shunted to micro environment to the area adjacent to the cell producing it. Cancer cells are favoured by acid inflammatory environment which leads to their faster growth and division, and accelerated disease progression. In addition, the cancer cells also produce ROS molecules, which, in turn damages the already dysfunctional mitochondria which further Leeds to disruption of cell function and progression of the cancerous environment.

"Cancer cell ferment a lot of glucose much more than what a normal cell could do because the rate of glycolysis is 10 to 15 times more than the rate of a normal cell."

Dr. Seyfried, in his paper published in the journal frontiers in "the cell and development biology", described the research involving nuclear cytoplasm transfer experiments. In this experiment he created cybrids by:

1. Transferring normal nuclei into cells containing cytoplasm that displayed warburg effect (excessive fermentation of glucose). They also replicated but majority of them did not survive!

2. Transferring nuclei of tumor cells into cells with normal cytoplasm, and the result was that the cell that replicated did survive, despite having nucleus with mutated DNA.

According to Dr. Seyfried, "in summary the information presented here supports the notation that cancer originates from damage to the mitochondria in the cytoplasm rather than from the damage to the genome in the nucleus".

Defective or uncontrolled inflammatory response: as one of the causes of cancer.

Inflammatory response is a fundamental function of immune system which kills bacteria entering our body. When it is working properly our immune system can bring back our body to normal in case of any disease like fever cough or cold. But when it isn't working it keeps on producing an inflammatory protein called cytokines which are essential for immune defences as they activate that help target invaders for destruction. Overproduction of cytokines can we can our immune system leading to chronic inflammation and drive cancer.

Immune surveillance is a way of body to destroy its own damaged cells. Some cells mutate and adapt the characteristics that allow then to escape from this surveillance. Cancer cells then even mutate more to progress and cause a full-blown cancer. All cancer cells take advantage of mutation and escape from immune system, start spreading in the location distant from their place of origin causing higher degree of inflammation and harder to restore balance.

"Fusion hybrid" hypothesis of cancer cell metastasis, takes the process a step further with the assumption that infiltrating macrophages (type of immune cells) re-establish themselves in location for away from their place of origin and contributes to an inflammatory cascade that can lead to Rapid and uncontrollable progression of disease and regression of immune system. The more the white spread the disease is higher is the degree of inflammation and harder it is to restore balance.

THE TEN TERRAIN OF CANCER

The ten terrain elements (we call them the Terrain Ten) we have identified are the physiological and emotional human elements that require to be in balance, in order to pause and prevent the cancer process.

The Terrain Ten:

1. Modification in- Genetic, epigenetic, and nutrigenomic.

2. Maximizing Immune system.

3. Toxins burden management

4. Enhancing mental and emotional well-being.

5. Balance of blood sugar

6. Changing inflammation and oxidative stress

7. Enhancement of circulation of blood, while inhibiting both angiogenesis and metastasis

8. Establishing balance in hormone

9. Rearranging stress levels and biorhythms

10. Balancing the microbiome.

All the 10 trains are however connected to each other. If, one is disrupted it might negatively affect all the others. For example, high stress levels leads to hormonal and blood sugar in balance and in turn high blood sugar level suppresses immune system. Cancel can capitalise on imbalances found within one of the ten train element. A tumor is nearly a side effect that occurs when a person's terrain is out of balance. Cancer does not just shows up easily in diagnosis rather it's a messenger telling you that some element regarding your emotional spiritual physical on metabolic- is not in harmony.

NOTES: Cancel is not just a single disease, it is a group of metabolic this functions which result in tumor. By this chapter you might have understood that cancer is not just uncontrollable growth of cells but also an indication of something wrong going on in your body.

CHAPTER 2

Is glucose being the reason for fluoride proliferation of cancerous cell? The science behind keto diet-

Yes. We all have cancer cells in our body it just requires a push to turn into to a dangerous uncontrollable dividing mass of cells and this push is given by glucose! As you know tumor is a group of cell having uncontrollable growth, increase amount of glucose in cells blue helps to proliferate the cancerous cell. See how it does!

As we read previously that glycolysis in Cancerous cells is much more than the rate of a normal cell. Therefore, the cells require more amount of glucose supply to compensate the rate of glycolysis. They increase the amount of glucose Transporter and insulin receptors in cell surface to increase the rate of glycolysis.

In 1922, Braunstein noted that glucose was absent from the urine of a diabetic patient after he was diagnosed with cancer. He suggested that the glucose is recruited to cancerous area where uh it is consumed at a higher rate than normal.

Nobel laureate Otto Warburg conducted many in vitro and animal experiments demonstrating that cancer cells thrive on glycolysis and produce high lactate levels even in the presence of abundant oxygen. He named this effect as Warburg effect.

MECHANISM

Glucose stimulates Beta cells of pancreas to release insulin which in turn allows glucose to enter the cell and produce energy. Insulin is secreted in a high amount in person taking high carbohydrate diet which in turn promotes the interaction of growth hormone receptor and growth hormone to produce "insulin like growth factor 1" in the liver hence promoting growth and proliferation of cells which can be harmful for cancer patients.

When hexokinase (the rate limiting enzyme of glycolysis) is over expressed it translocates from cytosol to the outer mitochondrial membrane where it interacts with voltage dependent anions channels and can disrupt caspase dependent cytochrome release which is responsible for apoptotic pathway of Cancer cells and make the cancer more resistant to chemotherapy.

HOW DOES CANCER CELLS ARE FLOURISH WITH THE HELP OF GLUCOSE AND GLUTAMINE?

Cancer cells thrive on fermentation products because they have dysfunctional mitochondria and possibly electron transport chain defects, which disrupt the normal adenosine triphosphate (ATP) production in mitochondria therefore the cancer cells heavily depend upon ATP produced from fermentation. A well-planned ketogenic diet can restrict cancer access to its fuel sources i.e., glucose and glutamine, while provides abundant energy to the Healthy cells.

In further chapters you will learn how ketogenic diet and other strategies stress the blooming of disease cells which restores the normal cellular signalling by their switching ability of changing metabolic dependence of fuel. The players in this molecular signalling pathway are- mTOR (mechanistic target of rapamycin), IGF-1 (insulin like growth factor, Type 1), Sirtuin 1, AMP- activated protein kinase, and other that at this point in your journey Messy more like secret code Dena diet about come. It is not important to understand these entire pathways to get benefits from keto diet.

ANOTHER FUEL DRIVING CANCER: GLUTAMINE

There is no question in any researcher's mind that cancer cells use glutamine as a source of energy allowing cancer cells to survive and thrive even in low oxygen condition. When the disease progress healthy cells are often destroyed by their cancerous neighbours self in order to meet their increased demand for glutamine. Although this problem can't be addressed by diet alone there are some actions you can take to cut down glutamine intake. You can refer to the nutritional labels for glutamine content in foods.

WHAT GOES WRONG WITH GLUCOSE METABOLISM?

We know that it is important to eat for survival but it is not necessary that only one type of food is necessarily required in an ideal diet. There is no single diet which fits best for everyone's needs. A cell is a complex organisation of cellular organelles which performs different functions and requires different nutrients for their working. Food can change the expression of some genes at cellular level - for example, Lac Operon model works in the presence of lactose which week we get from food.

Cancer is a game changer even if you feel that you are eating healthy food it might harm your system to cause cancer. Fermentation of glucose fuels cancer cells to grow. When Glucose level is high in your blood stream Beta cells in the pancreas begin to pump out insulin which helps to move glucose from Blood stream into the cells. Glucose molecules require Transporter proteins to facilitate their movement across the cell membrane and many of these proteins are activated by insulin. There are two transporters namely GLUT 1 and GLUT 3, found in brain tissues which are not dependent on presence of insulin for transporting glucose molecules into the cell.

Cancer cells have up to 10 times the normal number of insulin receptors in their cell membrane. Levels of the hormone IGF-1 (associated with cancer progression) rise along with insulin. IGF-1 can wind with the same receptors as insulin and cause a similar effect thereby contributing to the pro-cancer molecular activity in the cancer cells. This is harmful for our system!

Once the glucose molecule reach into the cytoplasm of the cell it splits up into 2 molecules of pyruvate in a process called glycolysis. In a normal cell most of the pyruvate passes into cell mitochondria where it gets oxidized to produce energy. In Cancer cells the mitochondria are damaged and cannot efficiently oxidize pyruvate to produce energy; more pyruvate remains in the cytoplasm where it gets fermented instead of getting oxidized.

Fermentation produces lactic acid or lactate which threatens the cells survival; therefore it is transported out of the cell where it acidifies the surrounding micro environment. This acidification causes inflammation which is a major promoter of cancer! Most of the lactate then goes to liver where it is converted back into glucose and returned to the bloodstream. This is an example of how changes at cellular level including alteration in genetic expression can control both the number of glucose Transporters on cell membrane and the amount of glucose that that's processed by fermentation in the cytoplasm versus oxidation in the mitochondria.

NOTES:

This chapter is all about how cancer cells depend on glucose for their growth and what happens if something is dysfunctional at cellular level? Hair it is thrown that a combination of genetic mutation and type of food can together be the cause of cancer. We cannot cure the genetic defect, but we can stop the duet of nutrition and genetic mutation from causing disease.

REFERENCE:

CHAPTER 3

What Causes Cancer?

Identifying the exact cause of cancer has proven tricky for scientists. After all, if we knew the cause, we'd be closer to finding a cure. However, a wealth of scientific research suggests a specific set of risk factors for the disease. Today, practically everyone knows that smoking cigarettes is linked to an increased risk of developing lung cancer, but how many know that there is more than thirty different factors that can lead to cancer? They can be grouped into three basic categories: infections (bugs), toxins, and biological factors. All of these things may cause cancer by disrupting the body's homeostasis, research suggests. One way they do this is by creating oxidative stress and inflammation. Inflammation and free radicals damage the RNA and DNA (the genetic material) inside the cells and with that, the cells' mitochondria, or energy-producing furnaces.

When the mitochondria are damaged and a cell can no longer efficiently produce energy for itself, it reverts to an inefficient method of energy production called glycolysis, in which it depends on sugar as a fuel source. In this state, the organs and body systems can no longer work properly. This leads to more DNA damage, less energy for normal cells, and more fuel for cancer cells.

- **Environmental Toxins.**

Environmental toxins are one of the biggest causes of DNA damage and cellular mutations. The following is a list of some toxins that research links to cancer. I have divided them into two categories. The first describes toxins you are probably aware of and which you may already know can cause cancer. The second describes toxins that you may have heard of, but which you may not know are associated with cancer.

The "Usual" Suspects

- Tobacco and smoking
- Mercury toxicity
- Sunlight—the shortwave rays of the sun cause reddening and sunburn and damage the superficial epidermal layers of the skin.

- **Other Toxins**

- Electromagnetic fields—Excessive exposure to electromagnetic field can cause cellular mutations that may lead to cancer.
- Geopathic stress—this comes from energies with the Earth that are created by underground cavitations, streams, and other geological features. Such energies are harmful to the body.
- Food additives—these include things such as stabilizers, food colouring, dyes, and artificial sweeteners.
- Foci infection, especially dental infection—many of us have hidden foci infections in the body, which are concentrated and localized pockets of infection that don't show up on routine lab tests. Among the most insidious and damaging of these are infections that are found in the mouth, and which are produced by root canals and jawbone infections. These infections produce toxins that could lead to inflammation and cancer.
- Immunosuppressive and other drugs
- Industrial toxins—these are ubiquitous in our air, food, and water supply. Industrial toxins, such as ammonia, fluoride, and chlorine, can be found in recycled water/tap water.

- Ionizing radiation—this comes from such tests as X-rays and CT scans. Radiation can increase an individual's cancer risk.

- Irradiated food—some of our food supplies, especially spices, fruits, and meat, is irradiated to eliminate organisms that cause food borne illness and to preserve the shelf life of food. This radiation damages the body. Although irradiated foods are common and found almost everywhere, there are clear ways to avoid them, such as buying produce from farmers' markets, asking whether your produce contain GMOs, and growing your own fruits and vegetables.

- Nuclear radiation—this comes from power plant accidents, such as what happened at the Fukushima power plant in 2011 in Japan.

- Pesticides—these are sprayed on fruits and vegetables to keep pathogens from destroying them.

- Polluted water—Tap water may contain such things as chlorine, fluorine, pharmaceutical drugs, and other chemicals linked to cancer.

- "Sick building" syndrome—this is caused by buildings that are contaminated by mould and other bio toxins.

- Xenoestrogens—these come from plastics and other chemical compounds that mimic the effects of human estrogens upon the body.

As you can see, there are many more environmental toxins and factors that are linked to cancer than what you may have been aware of!

Infections: Viruses, Bacteria, Parasites, and Fungi

Viruses, bacteria, parasites, and fungi, such as molds, mildews, and Candida, cause inflammation in the body and can increase cancer risk. Certain infections have also been directly linked to specific types of cancer. You may not always know whether you have an infection in your body that's creating an environment that is favorable to the development of cancer. A good integrative doctor can help you identify and eliminate any low-grade or underlying acute and chronic infections. Treating infections can help to lower your risk of any cancers that may be directly caused by those infections.

- **Biological Factors**

- A poor diet and nutritional deficiencies—much of our soil is nutrient-depleted and loaded with pesticides and other toxins, as are some of the foods that line our supermarket shelves. Also, many people don't consume whole foods and instead opt for processed, unhealthy, nutrient-depleted food.

- Toxic emotions and chronic stress—we describe stress and emotions in greater detail later in this book. Experimental studies have shown that stress can affect a tumor's ability to grow and spread.[7]

- Depressed thyroid function—this can result from gluten allergies, heavy metal toxins, radiation exposure, fluoride consumption, iodine deficiencies, and autoimmune disease, among other factors.

- Intestinal toxicity—Many of us have an unhealthy gastrointestinal tract due to infections or because we eat harmful foods. Some antibiotics, pesticides, environmental contaminants, pathogenic infections and other factors, damage beneficial bacteria and the mucosa of the stomach and intestines.

- Unbalanced "cellular terrain"—the internal terrain of your body determines how well every cell is oxygenated and nourished. Pathogens grow in the body when its internal terrain is out of balance. Nutritional imbalances, toxins, and acidic waste also contribute to an unhealthy terrain.

- Hormone therapies—Birth control pills, synthetic estrogen hormone replacement therapy, and hormone blockers disrupt the body's hormones and cause biochemical imbalances that may lead to cancer. A synthetic hormone found in conventionally processed meat and dairy products can also cause imbalances.

- Compromised detoxification—your body's ability to remove toxins can be compromised by bad circulation, scars, and other factors.

- Cellular oxygen deficiency—this is caused by excessive acidity in the body, as well as by a lack of exercise, pollution, and/or a lack of carbon dioxide in the cells.

According to American Medical Research LLC (AMR), a medical research company, toxins causes up to 75 percent of all cancers. Other infections including virus infection cause 20 to 25 percent of all cancers, and electromagnetic pollution and genetics are thought to cause less than 5 percent each of all cancers.

Otto Warburg, a Nobel Prize winner, German physician, and physiologist, discovered that cancer can occur when any cell is denied from 60 percent of its oxygen. Poor oxygenation results from a build-up of carcinogens and other toxins inside of and around the cells, which then damages the cell's ability to utilize oxygen. Additionally, psychological and emotional stress and nutritional imbalances are important contributing factors to cancer, although researchers aren't sure to what degree they play a role in its development. In The Cancer Revolution, I will show you how you can remove the effects of all of these factors from your body, so that you can either continue to live a cancer-free life, or help to fight a cancer you may already have.

Finally, the following are some additional facts about cancer that you may not know,

- Some studies link sugar to the growth of cancer cells. Sugar may increase the risk of certain types of cancer.

- A sedentary lifestyle creates a lack of oxygen in the body and can contribute to cancer growth.

- Bacteria, viruses, toxins, parasites, and heavy metals may indirectly increase cancer growth by suppressing the immune system.

- You are more likely to get cancer if your immune system is already compromised. According to the Canadian Cancer Society, a compromised immune system increases an individual's chances of contracting different viruses and bacteria that can increase the risk of cancer.

HOW IS A TUMOR FORMED?

Every cell can become a cancer cell under the favourable conditions. When a normal cell mutates, its normal functions gets damaged and it refrains to work as part of the team of other cells that it is a part of! It instead starts to work for itself and for its own survival by escaping from cell apoptosis. It starts growing rapidly and resists the body's natural cellular control mechanisms. So, tumors starts forming when a normal cell mutates into an "immortal," stubborn cancer cell. This cell then multiplies and proliferates until it becomes a mass of cells. Once this mass reaches a certain level, it seeks to form a "nest" somewhere in the body, and by this means it begins to establish itself in a specific organ or set of tissues to become what we know as a tumor.

As the tumor grows larger, it begins to require greater and greater amounts of nutrients from the blood, until it creates its own set of blood vessels and blood supply in a process called angiogenesis. Finally, if left unchecked, some of the cancer cells will break off from the tumor and establish new tumors, or "nests," in other parts of the body (metastasis).

Normally, your immune system will detect and destroy any cancer cells before they are able to form a colony of cells or a tumor. But if your immune system is compromised by toxins or infections, and is "blinded" by inflammation, cancer cells can more easily reproduce. As the cancer cells reproduce, they coat themselves with a substance called fibrin, which helps them hide from the immune system and stick together and form a colony. That colony will then attach to a wall in your smooth muscle and begin developing blood vessels so that it can get more nutrients from your blood to feed itself.

To further enable its survival, the newly developed tumor will send out a lot of other information, in signals known as growth factors, to the rest of the body that will aid in its growth and development. There are different signals that tumors put out, so it's important to prevent or halt these transmissions. Cancer has multiple survival strategies, all of which need to be addressed with different treatments, at the same time that your body must be repaired and restored from the "earthquake."

CAN WE PREVENT CANCER?

Although many factors in our environment cause cancer, and cancer has multiple survival mechanisms to help it grow in the body, most of the time we can prevent it! All humans have 75 million cancer cells in their body at any given time, our immune system keeps these cells in check, but when the immune system becomes compromised over a long period, these cells can begin to proliferate, or multiply. But we can help to stop this process by consuming a nutritious diet.

It generally takes ten to twelve years on for a single cancer cell to become a full-grown tumor in the body. This means you often have a lot of time to eliminate the things that are causing cancer, if you catch it in the early stages. There are early-detection tests that you can do, such as the Cancer Profile! This test, among others, aims to help determine whether the environment in your body is favourable to the development of cancer, or whether cancer is already "brewing or fermenting" somewhere in it, many years before it actually becomes a disease.

Currently, not many doctors in the United States know how to prevent cancer because most are trained to be reactive with their patients instead of proactive. The good news is that increasingly, doctors are being trained in functional and integrative medicine and are helping their patients help prevent cancer, just as we do at our clinic. Cancer is a global illness, affecting the entire body; it's not just a disease of a single body part, so it's essential that you work with a doctor who can look at your entire body and tell you whether you have an internal environment that is favourable to its development.

To prevent or fight cancer, you must also resolve the stress and emotional conflicts in your life. I often ask my patients whether they want to be well, and tell them, "I can't help you until you get your mind in order." You must want to be well and discipline yourself to do all the right things if you want to heal.

It's like weight loss. Unfortunately, according to the United Institute of Health and Human Services, about two-thirds (68.8%) of the population is characterized as being overweight. Some are overweight because they don't "pay attention to their intention" (their mind and thoughts). Everyone wants to pop a pill for every ill, but this doesn't work. So, why are we still looking to "pop a pill," when we know that doesn't work?

Another analogy I give my patients has to do with driving. I will say to them, "Do you drive? If you do, then you know that there is a rule book for driving, and that you have to know the rules and laws of driving a car." Then, I will ask them, "How many stop signs did you run today? None, right? Because you know that you'd probably get a ticket, hurt somebody, or crash the car if you did.

"Similarly, you have to pay attention to the rules of your body. Because nobody wants to get into a car accident, and I don't want you to have a body accident! If you follow the rules and laws of Mother Nature, then the right things will happen in your body."

It's not about perfection, though, because none of us are perfect drivers, and you aren't going to be a perfect driver with your health. But you want to follow the rules of nature so that your body works for you, not against you. What percentage of the time did you think you can get away with running a stop sign? Once in a while, right? But that's about it.

Preventing cancer doesn't need to be complicated. You just need to learn a few key things about how to be well, which you can do without spending a fortune. Likewise, if you have already been diagnosed with cancer, there are many simple lifestyles and dietary changes that you can make that can help you battle the disease and live a longer, more vibrant life, which you will find throughout this book.

HOW CANCER AFFECTS OUR BLOOD CIRCULATION?

In healthy adults, new blood vessels don't normally need to grow, with a few exceptions: the monthly growth of the uterine lining, which facilitates the menstrual cycle; pregnancy; and following an injury. And normally the body has a checkpoint system for regulating angiogenesis, a system comprising stimulators and inhibitors. When blood is needed, the body sends signals certain to some growth factors which include vascular endothelial growth factor, an angiogenesis stimulator, to make new vessels. TNF and IGF-1 are also able to stimulate the production of new blood vessels. Normally when vessels are no longer needed they are dissolved through the action of angiogenesis inhibitors. When these systems of checks and balances become dysregulated, however, cancer and other diseases can occur. Impaired blood vessel development results in arteriosclerosis and increased risk of stroke, while much blood vessels are a cause of pulmonary hypertension and endometriosis. Dozens of diseases in addition to cancer are linked to angiogenesis.

Cancer cells need a blood supply to grow and nourish their rapid metabolism. Like any organism, without food or oxygen they cannot survive. And any tumor that grows past a very small size (0.5–1 millimetre, approximately the size of the tip of a ballpoint pen) needs new blood. Like little vampires, tumor cells commandeer the normal process of angiogenesis for their own survival. Cancer cells are able to "switch on" angiogenesis and activate VEGF while at the same time deactivating angiogenesis inhibitors.

When microscopic cancers start out, they reach that ballpoint-pen size and then most cancers stop—a state called "cancer without disease." When the body is in balance, it doesn't provide blood supply to these tiny tumors, and they eventually die. But cancer cells get creative when they become hypoxic, meaning when they are deprived of oxygen. Hypoxia can occur when tumors grow and also with low blood pressure, chronic pulmonary disease (COPD), high altitude, and anemia. By activating a process called the hypoxia stress response, tumors emit signals to neighboring blood vessels, persuading them to throw them a "vessel extension lifeline" that will deliver needed oxygen and nutrients. Once cancer cells connect with new food and oxygen lifelines, not only do they grow, but they also like to travel. A growing tumor is rarely the main cause of death; it's when cancer metastasizes to a new location that it becomes a big problem.

That tumor "lifeline" formation is directed by VEGF, and therefore the majority of anti-angiogenesis drugs are VEGF inhibitors. The aim of angiogenesis inhibitors is to prevent the growth and migration of new blood vessels. Bevacizumab, an angiogenesis inhibitor we discussed previously, has been shown to slightly improve survival rates in different types of cancer, yet also indiscriminately cuts off circulation in other areas of the body with side effects, including bowel perforations, and hemorrhaging.

According to Chinese medicine, stagnant blood, or what Western doctors call "sticky" blood, is one of the main causes of cancer. With blood stagnation, nutrients from the blood do not enter cells efficiently, cellular waste is not properly removed, and cells, basically, become sick. No milk delivery, no trash pickup. The term viscosity refers to the thickness and stickiness of a liquid. In the case of blood, its viscosity is directly correlated with its ability to flow through vessels. Blood should flow through our bodies like a river. When the river gets dammed up or filled with debris and flow stops, then all sorts of things can grow. Think of the difference between a mud puddle and a clear stream. Over time, stagnant water becomes host for all sorts of pathogens and bacteria. In the case of cancer, after cachexia and infection, circulation issues are the cause of death in cancer patients. Considering heart disease has been the number one killer in the United States for decades (though quickly being overtaken by cancer), we clearly have rampant circulation issues that are linked—unquestionably—to diet and lifestyle.

Blood that is sticky or stagnant means that it is more prone to clotting, or coagulating. Here is how that process works: Within a moment of getting a cut, for example, damaged skin tissue will activate platelets within the blood in the torn blood vessel—perhaps a vein or even an artery—to become sticky and to clump together like glue around the cut, forming a clot at the damaged part of the blood vessel. (Platelets, also called thrombocytes, are components of the blood that helps it clots and are produced in the bone marrow.) Soon threadlike proteins called fibrin, arrive to form structural scaffolding throughout the clot to hold it in place (we will talk more about them in a minute).

Thrombocytosis is a condition of having too many platelets. It can increase risk of either spontaneous blood clotting or bleeding, depending on what is causing it. Cancer and coagulation activation go hand in hand. Cancerous tumors can activate platelets, which help them to both grow and spread. These activated platelets form around tumors, shielding them from immune cells and also from chemotherapy drugs. Activated platelets also assist in metastasis and migration by creating pathways into the bloodstream and promoting angiogenesis. Again, a normal bodily process is hijacked and subverted by cancer cells.

Hypercoagulation also increases the production of fibrins, the structural proteins that help with clotting. Fibrin is formed from fibrinogen (a protein produced by the liver). When tissue gets damaged, it results in bleeding, and then fibrinogen is converted into fibrin by the action of the enzyme thrombin. The drug heparin is an anticoagulant (or blood thinner), which works through a multistep pathway by preventing the conversion of fibrinogen to fibrin. Heparin is useful in treating and preventing blood clots in veins, arteries, and the lung and also decreases the spread of cancer; it works so well that Dr.Nasha actually considers it an underutilized antimetastatic pharmaceutical!

A high fibrinogen level indicates sticky blood and has been linked to reduced survival and poor response to treatments in certain cancers. Foods with a higher glycemic index, including sugars, are known to be associated with elevated fibrinogen. Thus, one natural antigen to high fibrinogen is the elimination of sugar from the diet, and another is consuming coumarin-containing plants and herbs. Coumarin is a sweet-smelling compound found in aniseed, cassia cinnamon, dandelion, horseradish, and wild lettuce. Coumarin is used in topically in perfumes, but when ingested it has anticoagulant properties.

NOTES:

To know about cancer, you first have to understand the cause of it. Though cancer cells thrive on glucose, but it requires a kick start to grow uncontrollably and form tumor. This kick start is given by my agents who can cause mutation. The cause of cancer you might be suffering from cannot be generally predicted. There are many causes which are unknowingly included in our day to day life that might cause cancer. By having a grip on all possible ways which might cause mutation, you can protect yourself from them.

CHAPTER 4

Is keto a way of fasting to starve cancer cells?

Ketogenic diet is much more than just Starving cancer cells for glucose! Our body has the ability to handle a number of toxins through activation of a healthy adaptive response known as *hormesis.* The concept of hormesis is, "that which does not kill us makes us stronger", it is a Friedrich Nietzsche's quotation. The study of hormesis is has health implications which is beyond the scope of this book. It has become a very active area of research in health healthy aging community. Latest see how this quotation of starving helps to crave cancer.

Benefits of fasting

Glucose and insulin levels reduce in all forms of fasting, and we become more insulin sensitive. It results in lowered activity of IGF-1, a hormone associated with cell proliferation in many cancers. While fasting our cells find a way to cut down energy requirement in the areas where it is required the most like for cell growth and proliferation. They also break down activities by removing accumulated garbage and recycling it into new building materials. This housekeeping is called autophagy; it is an activity directed at replacing mitochondria. In this process old damaged or inefficient cell organelles are killed for good. This also includes digesting of dysfunctional Mitochondria found in Cancer cells.

Mitochondrion is an important organelle for energy production, but also a role in directing cell activities such as apoptosis (cell suicide). They control cell signalling Pathways (such as mTOR) that are involved in Cancer progression and pathway that help in inhibiting Cancer (pathway such as AMPK). The metabolic theory of cancer represents that is functional mitochondria are the root cause of initiation and progression of Cancer cells.

Calorie restriction is the main goal of fasting. Since you go fasting, it is important that you keep meeting your essential nutrients while having food. There are many benefits of restricting calories regarding dealing the chronic diseases associated with aging and also so in dealing with cancer. Following is some benefits you will achieve by restricting your calorie intake:

- **Inhibition of angiogenesis:**

Cancer cells direct the development of new blood vessels to supply blood to them. This new blood vessel networks increase the supply of nutrients to cancer cells. It is well-documented that restricting calorie intake can suppress angiogenesis.

- **Reduces chronic inflammation**

Calorie restriction reduces chronic inflammation and also improves outcome in type 2 diabetes, hypertension, osteoarthritis and coronary heart disease stroke.

- **Enhances apoptosis**

Failure of apoptosis is one of the Hallmarks of cancer. As you read above that during fasting yourself fine done easy way to cut down calorie consumption so it digests its own old and dysfunctional cell organelles for good.

- **Limit the availability of nutrients**

As you have read that cancer cells thrive on glucose, fasting can inhibit opportunities for cancer cell to feed on nutrients for proliferation.

- **Increases lifespan**

Beyond cancer, calorie restriction has been shown to extend health and life span of variety of organisms ranging from yeast to primates.

- **Enhancement of autophagy**

It enhances a cellular housekeeping process known as autophagy which kills the dysfunctional cells and restore healthy cellular signalling.

FEW THINGS TO KNOW BEFORE FASTING:

Identify the situations noted below, and take steps for fasting according to it. Seek help for from your Healthcare team before you decide to fast.

- If you had a problem of sluggish gallbladder or any other gallbladder disease- water only fast may make your situation worse! Here there is more risk than benefits of fasting.
- If you are an older adult who is inactive cancer treatment or not yet recovered from the effects of surgery of cancer therapies, you should not fast for more than 48 hours. It will cause you too much stress on your system and lead to breakdown instead of repair.
- If you have history of eating disorder you might have a potential pitfall of slipping into a pattern of feasting and fasting that is actually closer to bingeing and purging.
- Don't fall prey to every e post from your favourite blogger. Although they may hold strong opinions but it is better to be verified by scientific evidence.

Types of fasting:

- **Intermittent and short term fast**

These fasts are for 2 to 3 days with meals in regular time after a prolonged day of fasting. Like in Ramadan you fast for 30 days irregularly by doing- no water and no food fasting from Sunrise to sunset. After that in the evening you can eat it whatever you want but that should be keto food.

- **Water only fasts**

Many people try to start ketogenic diet with water only fast lasting for 2 to 3 days. This can be very difficult since you are jumping from Reliance on glucose to the new metabolism of ketosis. Those who are already Keto adapted can also opt for two to three days water only fast periodically.

- **Protein sparing modified fasts**

It is not an actual fasting because here you take a good amount of protein. It is popular with some people because they tend to lose weight and gain lean body mass. However, this is not a good choice for most people with cancer because excess protein made drive disease progression (as excess of protein is converted into carbohydrates)

- **Extended fast**

This proof that long fast remote autophagy at a greater rate it helps the body to clear out all the diseased cells and cellular organelles like dysfunctional mitochondria. However long fast are very stressful on mind and body and not appropriate for you right now and also you will lose weight with muscle mass.

WHICH IS THE MOST ADAPTABLE FASTING?

Fasting all day long for 2 to 3 days can be difficult for some persons so the best way to fast is short term fasting and intermittent fasting.

- **Intermittent fasting**

Recent research has been done on both humans and animals to see the effects of fasting. They are testing a range of hypothesis that attempt to identify both the benefits and risks of different modified fasting protocols. This introduces a whole host of variables that sets base for new researche. In the journal *PLoS ONE*, research on energy restriction in animal model of cancer reviewed that ketogenic diet show improved outcomes whereas intermittent fasting did not appear to have any impact. Nevertheless, intermittent fasting is an add-on therapy to either calorie restriction or a ketogenic diet. This study also applies on humans and not only on the animal models.

Many variations of intermittent fasting

"Fasting" means many things to many people. Have a closer look at the many variations?

- Alternate-day fasting (including variations that allow for 20 percent of normal calorie intake on fasting days alternating with a 20 percent increase in calorie consumption on non-fasting days).
- 48-hour cycles of fasting (water only)
- One day per week of water-only fasting
- 5:2 (5 days of normal eating; 2 days of modified fasting, such as 20 percent of normal caloric intake)

- "Time-restricted feeding," a scientific but awkward name used to describe daily fasting with varying "windows" of eating hours versus fasting hours.

fasting

Nausea and vomiting associated with drug therapy make it difficult to consume any food other than drinks. Drinks are mostly loaded with easily digestible carbs and added sugar. This is obviously a huge problem if you are following ketogenic diet. So, short term fasting during chemotherapy can reduce both the number and variety of treatment related side effects. Short term fasting also protects normal cell from damage and sterilizes cancer cells to drug therapies enhancing the therapy efficiency. If, you don't feel hungry it is better not to eat anything! Whenever you are going for chemotherapy, try to remain under the watchful eyes of a dedicated caregiver.

Patients who are going under chemotherapy are very surprised to realise that how easy it is to not eat when they are in ketosis. This is because ketosis adapts the body in such a way that it does not rely on dietary fuel supplement to produce energy rather it makes energy from stored fat in your body without making you feel hungry. Therefore, it is easy to skip food while chemotherapy.

Basic of short term fasting during chemotherapy

- Stop eating 12 to 24 hours before treatment.
- Fast the day of the treatment.
- Resume eating the following day.
- Stay hydrated! Water protects the kidneys and helps flush out toxins.
- Some people may choose to drink soothing bone broth (modified fasting!).

NOTES:

Fasting has been practiced since ages to cure many diseases. It was easy for people to fast 500 years ago because of scarcity of food and difficulty to fetch them. Now days where there is plenty food items available around you it becomes hard to restrict yourself from eating them. Make a mind set of living healthy and set your fasting goal shot and strong for like 2 to 3 days intermittent fasting.

REFERENCE:

CHAPTER 5

What is ketogenic diet?

Don't ketogenic is derived from two words which means Ketone and generic which means to produce. In this diet ketones are produced in our body. The purpose of this diet is to make the body enter into nutritional state referred as ketosis where the body produces and burns ketones for energy. Ketogenic diet contains very less carbohydrate moderate protein and high fat diet. This diet burns fat for energy rather than carbohydrates. In our body carbohydrates eventually breaks down into glucose molecules true provide energy in the extra amount of glucose which is not utilized for producing energy is converted into 2 fat molecules to be stored in the body. However, if we cut down the amount of carbohydrate ingestion we will be cutting down fats into 2 fatty acids and Ketone bodies which will be used as a source of energy in place of glucose.

"In this diet your body starts reversing everything that it has been doing to store fat."

PROCESS OF KETOSIS-

- Insulin hormone helps the body to utilise glucose as a source of energy. Moreover, with reduced carb intake, the blood sugar level reduces and the amount of insulin produced by the body also decreases. Instead the body produces more glucagon a hormone that triggers the liver to start metabolizing stored glycogen from the liver and muscle cells

- In the same time body produce human growth hormone and along with glucagon it triggers the release of fats from stored area around the body after which these fats are transported to the liver. These fats are then broken down in the liver cells to produce fatty acids and glycerol. This fatty acid then goes through a series of process to produce Ketone bodies which is used as a fuel instead of glucose.

- As the body convert more fats into fatty acids and glycerol more amount of Ketone bodies are produced. Once the amount of ketone out numbers the molecules of glucose our body starts to use that Ketone body as a source of energy. This is referred to as nutritional ketosis and sets in when the level of Ketone concentration in blood stream is 1.5-3 mmol/L.

For this to take place you should take-
20-30 gm of carbohydrates per day
1.5-2.6 per pound of your weight
65-75 percent of your calorie should come from fats (healthy fats)

WHAT IS THE REASON BEHIND CONSUMING LOT OF FATS?

The reason behind eating lot of fats is to give your body enough energy without increasing carbohydrate consumption. This is a great impact on metabolism as fats do not trigger the production of insulin. As for your knowledge you should know that insulin hormone hinders fat metabolism. Also, fats tend to be feeling and digests slowly e which helps to keep you away from craving. This phenomenon can greatly help in the process of weight loss.

WHY SHOULD YOU TAKE PROTEIN IN A MODERATE QUANTITY?

The reason why you should take a moderate amount of protein is to avoid the chance of body converting any excess protein into carbohydrates. Process in which protein is converted into carbohydrates is called gluconeogenesis. The amount of protein you take should be just enough for muscle repair and maintenance.

The concept of ketogenic diet is that it takes advantage of your body's natural system of utilizing fat for fuel. By switching to a low carbohydrate diet your body at that and becomes unavailable to utilize the readily available source of carbohydrate that was once available to it before you started your keto diet. Instead, it begins to use both existing and new stored fats have its source of energy which helps in weight loss by reducing the amount of stored fat.

IS KETOGENIC DIET HELPFUL- ONLY IN WEIGHT LOSS?

Keto diet is the alternative way of fasting without Starving yourself. As you know it utilises your body fat instead of glucose to produce energy and helps you in weight loss, it also has other benefits health benefits which are results of deprivation of blood glucose level. The following are the health benefits which you will receive by following keto diet-

- Reduces your appetite and unnecessary cravings

One of the main reasons for people to gain weight is their inability to control their huge appetite and small cravings for a calorie rich foods on which day feed on for several times in a day. By adapting to ketogenic diet you can reduce your appetite and unnecessary cravings which makes you feel hungry 24/7. Studies have shown that when you to cut down carb intake you will start eating less with time.

- Trim down the stubborn belly fat

Visceral fat is the fat lying around your abdominal cavity which starts surrounding your organs when it increases in size and quantity. It is the most difficult type of fat to get rid of. Having a large amount to visceral fat in your abdomen can result in inflammation metabolic dysfunction and insulin resistance. Keto diet helps in eliminating this visceral fat from abdomen giving it a slimmer shape and appearance

- Fights from heart diseases

Triglycerides refer to the fat molecules in our body which is approved by the studies that they have a close link with heart diseases. Excess amount of triglycerides in your body results in higher chances of you being vulnerable two heart diseases and high blood pressure. The major cause of increase in triglyceride concentration is the amount of carbohydrate consumed. Cut down your intake of Carbohydrate and you will be able to reduce the amount of triglycerides in your body which consequently decrease your chances of suffering from fatal cardiovascular conditions.

- Fights type 2 diabetes

In type 2 diabetes your body stop responding to insulin becoming insulin resistance. Insulin is a hormone which converts excess of glucose in blood which are not utilised for making energy e into glucagon. Your body often becomes resistant to insulin when there is an enormous amount of glucose in your body. Therefore, if you eat fewer carbohydrates you will be able to eliminate the probability of developing insulin resistant condition and reduce your risk of becoming type 2 diabetic patients. Therefore, in keto diet where there is a very less amount of carbohydrate will prevent you from suffering from this disease.

- Reduce chances of having high blood pressure

As you read above that triglyceride is one of the reasons of heart diseases and high blood pressure, switching to low carbohydrate diet can reduce your chances of suffering from high blood pressure and related problems. Studies have also shown that half of the people who follow a low carbohydrate diet had their blood pressure level reduced greatly. One of the reasons for this can also be because you end up losing weight on a ketogenic diet and studies have shown a close relationship between weight loss and reduction in blood pressure.

- Promotes the production of HDL

HDL is also known as high density lipoprotein or good cholesterol. It is a lipoprotein that carries cholesterol in your blood. LDL for low density lipoprotein which is also called bad cholesterol is responsible for carrying cholesterol from your liver to body parts HDL takes the cholesterol from blood to liver so that it can be either excreted or reused. Fats contain high density lipoprotein and carbohydrates contain low density lipoprotein therefore by eating a diet rich in fats and low in carbs will help you to promote the production of HDL and with the increase level of HDL your chances of suffering from heart disease will decrease as well.

- Prevents proliferation of Cancer cells.

Cancer cells are the uncontrolled and fast dividing cells which require enormous amount of energy trips to proliferate. It is hard to burn fat for fuel therefore cancer cells depend on glucose for energy because glucose easily breakdown to produce ATP. Tumor cells require a large amount of glucose to live. So, by following keto diet you can reduce your blood Glucose level and the chance of Cancer cells to proliferate in your body.

NOTES:

Keto diet is a new nutritional therapeutic approach of starving cancer cells instead of starving yourself. It will help you to lose weight suppress hunger and sugar cravings. It ultimately leads you to a healthy life. Your meal plan should be based on the above calculations of carbohydrates, proteins and fats for making a right diet chart.

REFERENCE:

CHAPTER 6

What is important for a keto diet?
1. Medical fitness

As you know keto diet alters your metabolic dependence of energy, you might experience some side effects. Initially you will experience some weight loss followed by a plateau (a condition in which weight loss stops). Don't get worried about the plateau condition and follow the tips mentioned to overcome it.

People with following metabolic conditions should not follow this diet-

- Type 1 Diabetes
- Beta oxidation defects
- Primary carnitine deficiency
- Pyruvate carboxylase deficiency
- Carnitine translocase deficiency
- Carnitine palmitoyl transferase (CPT) Type 1 & 2 deficiency
- Porphyria

People with following medical conditions should avoid keto diet-

- Malnutrition
- Gastric bypass surgery
- Impaired liver function
- Gallbladder disease
- Kidney failure

- Pancreatitis
- Abdominal tumors
- Impaired gastric motility
- If you are pregnant or breastfeeding

2. Right food
➢ **What to eat?**

FATS -
- Beef
- Butter
- Chicken
- Duck Fat
- Ghee
- Mayonnaise
- Olive Oil
- Sesame Oil
- Coconut Oil

PROTEINS -

- Lamb
- Goat
- Pork
- Chicken
- Turkey
- Duck
- Goose
- Anchovies
- Calamari
- Lobster
- Catfish
- Sardines
- Snapper
- Tuna
- Clams
- Salmon
- Crab
- Tofu
- Shrimp
- Mussels
- Oysters
- Peanut Butter

- Squid

VEGETABLES -

- Bean
- Asparagus
- Escarole
- Bell peppers *
- Fennel
- Bamboo shoots
- Beet
- Broccoli
- Avocado
- Carrots *
- Celery
- Garlic
- Spinach
- Zucchini
- Scallions
- Mushrooms
- Shallots
- Onions *
- Radishes
- Sauerkraut
- Tomatoes *
- Turnips

*high carb content! Therefore, they should be consumed in a limited amount.

DAIRY PRODUCTS -

- Yogurt
- Sour cream
- Monterey Jack
- whipping cream
- Farmer cheese
- Cheddar cheese
- Swiss cheese
- Colby
- Cream cheese
- Munster
- Cottage cheese
- Blue cheese
- Provolone cheese
- Marscapone cheese

NUTS & SEEDS -

It is recommended to soak the nuts and seeds to get rid of any anti-nutrients they might be present in it. They have very high carbs content; therefore, you will need to limit your intake. Do not fully depend upon them for all of your protein requirements because too much intake of them can cause increased inflammation. They can also cause a disturbance in you moods.

- Walnuts
- Sunflower seeds
- Hemp seeds
- Almonds
- Pistachios
- Chestnuts
- Peanuts
- Sesame seeds
- Cashews

BEVERAGES –

Make sure that all beverages you drink - should be free of sugar. You can use artificial sweeteners in a very little amount. Your all beverages should be decaffeinated because caffeine can possibly increase blood sugar level.

- Coffee and tea (decaffeinated)
- Lime juice
- Hemp milk
- Coconut milk
- Hazelnut milk
- Bone broth
- Flavoured water
- Soy milk
- Herbal tea
- Almond milk
- Cashew milk

FRUITS, SPICES & MISCELLANEOUS

Most fruits contain a high amount of carbohydrates in the form of fructose, so they should be mostly avoided, but, there are certain berries which can be enjoyed in small once in a while in small amounts.

- Blackberries
- Cranberries
- Raspberries
- Blueberries
- Strawberries

SPICES

The spices will be your secret weapons as you navigate the keto diet. Most are very low in carbohydrates and rich in flavour. The net carbohydrate information for major spices per tablespoon follows.

- Allspice, ground, 3g
- Basil, dried, 0.9g
- Black pepper, 2.4g
- Cayenne pepper, 1.6g
- Cinnamon, 1.7g
- Cloves, 1.7g
- Cumin, ground, 2.1g
- Curry powder, 1.6g
- Garlic powder, 5.3g
- Nutmeg, 2g
- Oregano, ground, 0.4g
- Onion powder, 5.2g
- Paprika, 1.2g
- Pumpkin pie spice, 3.1g
- Sage, ground, 0.4g
- Tarragon, ground, 2g
- Thyme, ground, 1.1g
- Ginger, ground, 3.1g
- Vanilla extract, imitation, 0.3g

- Parsley, dried, 0.3g
- Vanilla extract, pure, 1.6g
- White pepper, 3g

➢ FOODS TO AVOID ABSOLUTELY -
Sugars & Sweeteners

- Barley malt
- Fruit syrups
- Cane juice
- Malt syrup
- Confectioner's sugar
- Maple syrup
- Caramel
- Rice syrup
- Beet sugar
- Maltodextrin
- Fruit juice concentrate
- White sugar
- Corn syrup
- Molasses
- Coconut sugar
- Maltose
- Sorghum
- Brown sugar

- Date sugar

GRAINS & GRAIN PRODUCTS

- Rice
- Wheat
- Rye
- Barley
- Sorghum
- Tricale
- Oats
- Bread
- Muffins
- Tortillas
- Pancakes
- Cookies
- Tarts
- Oatmeal
- Cakes
- Cream of wheat
- Corn chips
- Popcorn

FRUITS, VEGETABLES & LEGUMES

- Bananas
- Apples
- Pears
- Grapefruits
- Oranges
- Peaches
- Watermelon
- Honeydew Melon
- Cherries
- Gooseberries
- Figs
- Grapes
- Mango
- Guava
- Kiwi
- Plums
- Papaya
- Pineapple
- Potatoes
- Pomegranates
- Sweet potatoes

ENRIC SCOTT

- Okra
- Peas
- Kidney beans
- Chickpeas
- Black beans
- Lentils

OTHER FOODS TO AVOID -

- Canned stews
- Canned soups
- Foods labelled as - 'low-carb', 'low-fat', 'sugar-free'.
- Processed, boxed food
- Beer
- Dessert wines; dry wines, to be taken in limited amounts
- Hard liquor
- Carbonated drinks
- Milk; liquid milk contains lactose.

3. Right plan.

Every individual's diet plan suits their own schedule, so make a personal plan to approach your fitness journey. When, you start ketogenic diet you should have a well planned diet chart and recipes to suit your taste and to count the daily calorie intake. It is very easy to slip back into poor eating habits so, the key to develop healthy lifestyle is to plan a consistent and well balanced meal plan for every week in advance. Here is a weekly meal plan which will help you to organise you're your diet of 30 days.

WEEK 1:

The first week of your ketogenic diet is going to be the hardest because; it will be the basic transition week, therefore, you need to keep it simple and convenient as possible.

- Start your keto diet on the weekend because you will have plenty of time to devote yourself in making new meals according to the plan. On weekends, you will be stress free and you will be able to focus on starting keto diet.
- Choose few recipes and prepare for 5 to 6 different types of meal for the entire week. Calculate and make a list of the ratios of the ingredients which you will use in your recipe.
- **Breakfast-** you could eat eggs or any type of meat, vegetables, nuts and fruits which are allowed in the diet chart with a cup of black coffee or tea, without sugar.
- **Lunch-** your lunch should be heavy, containing high amount of fat. You can follow the recipes and give them a high fat dressing paired with a delicious salad.
- **Snacks-** kill your small cravings by a light and a small portion of keto snacks. You can snack on allowed nuts, vegetables, fruits and eggs.
- **Dinner-** your dinner should also be heavy, but, it should include more green and leafy vegetables.

There should not be any desert during the first week.

Keto flu- it is a condition where you will experience different side effects of keto diet. It is mainly characteristic by fogginess, fatigue and headache. You might feel sick and want to give up on the diet, but, you have to keep going to achieve your goals, because all this side effects are only temporary. Drink plenty of fluids throughout the day; it will help you to stay calm even during keto flu. Coconut water is a great alternative to beverages like tea and coffee. It is a diuretic drink, so you will urinate frequently.

WEEK 2:

Second week diet plan will be slightly little different from the first one because, you will introduce new recipes in this week.

- **Breakfast-** for this week, the only breakfast you will have is- "bulletproof coffee". Let me explain you what, is Bulletproof coffee- it contains tons of good fats, which can kick start your body every day and help transition to the keto fat burning status. It is made by butter or ghee and coconut oil or MCT oil mixed in toxin free coffee. This drink might sound disgusting to you, but it actually tastes good and is very much beneficial for keto diet.

The above-mentioned toxin free coffee means coffee which is free of toxins or lotoxane coffee. Look for light roasted coffee and not super dark roast because the dark it's roasted the more carcinogen it contains. Lightly roasted coffee contains a very low amount of carcinogen, and the naturally occurring antioxidants in the coffee actually cancel them out. Prefer wet processed coffee beans over dry processed coffee beans, as it does not allowed mould to grow in the coffee beans while being processed, so they naturally have fewer toxins. If, you pee a lot after drinking bullet proof coffee then it's perfectly normal because it contains coconut oil which is a diuretic substance.

- **Lunch-** lunch in the second week may be similar to that of first week. You can add some new dishes in this week but try to keep the portion similar to that of the first week. Generous portion of meat bathed in fat dressing paired with the salad will do well for your lunch.

- **Dinner**-dinner can be similar to the pattern of lunch. You can eat anything that's suggested to recipes. There should be no desert in this week also but don't worry you can have it from the third week.

WEEK 3:

At this week you, have completed your half way through the keto diet plan of 30 days. This week will be a little different and difficult than the first two weeks. You will be practicing intermittent fasting in between breakfast and dinner. When you first your body breaks down more fat to provide energy to your body resulting in more weight loss. However, fasting is a great technique to get rid of all the toxins residing in your body. In this week don't exhaust your body by doing intense exercises, rather do mild exercise take rest and have a plenty of sleep.

- **Breakfast-** this week breakfast you not only consume bullet proof coffee but a heavy amount of fat sources to keep you active throughout the 12 hours of fasting. Take a good amount of breakfast having large amount of back to keep useful and active. Do not forget to hide rate yourself with plenty of water or any alternative drink like coconut water.

- **Dinner-** after breakfast you directly move to dinner, so you are allowed to take whatever you want as per suggested in this book. You can also refer to keto recipes from others sources if you are running low on ideas. Keep yourself hydrated throughout the day, even at night.

- **Dessert-** after saying a strict no to desert- in first 2 weeks of the diet plan, this week you can have a portion of them. You can refer to the recipe suggested in this book which is dessert fat bomb and cheesecake. Always keep in mind, to eat the portion in less quantity.

WEEK 4:

This is the last week of your diet plan which is the toughest week and you will be fasting more; so be prepared.

- **No breakfast or lunch-** this week's plan is to finalize the weight loss effect on your body. Therefore, the main goal in this week is to do even more fasting. You will eat nothing until dinner time during the whole week. It is going to be hard but not impossible. Keep yourself hydrated throughout the day by drinking at least four litres of fluids. Water, tea and coffee are allowed, but no bulletproof coffee because it is diuretic in nature and can dehydrate you. You can also take green tea (it contains phenol that work as antioxidant and keep you energetic) which increases the rate of metabolism and fastens the rate of fat oxidation process by 15 percent.

- **Dinner-** dinner can be extremely lavish. You can double the amount of portion you ate in the previous week. It is suggested that when you break your fast- you should eat a small portion of snack and then jump to two big dinner portions after an hour or two. You can keep eating small desserts in this week as well.

Setting Up a Nontoxic Kitchen

The idea for this step is to create a kitchen space that is a not only easy to use and well-stocked, but also free of toxins. So once you've gotten all the unhealthy foods out, it's time to take a closer look at your systems, gadgets, storage options, and products. Food storage containers and products including plastic, such as Tupperware, plastic bags, and plastic wrap, can contain endocrine-disrupting chemicals like- BPA and other compounds that are carcinogenic. Consider switching to glass jars for food storage, using reusable bags for produce, and using aluminium foil rather than plastic wrap.

Next look under your sink at the cleaning products, they can be some of the most toxic products in your home. Ingredients including DEA, TEA, and 1, 4-dioxane in cleaners contribute to cancer and hormone disruption. Most household cleaning needs can be made safely with a scrubber sponge and ingredients like water, liquid castile soap, vinegar, lemon juice, essential oils, and baking soda for scrubbing greasy areas. At least look for products that indicate that they are plant-based and biodegradable.

Your pots and pans are next. Non-stick surfaces and metal pans coated with a synthetic polymer known as Teflon which are highly toxic. Toxic fumes released from these pots and pans at high temperatures are associated with smaller size in newborn babies, increased cholesterol levels, imbalanced thyroid hormone levels, liver inflammation, and weakening of immune defence against disease. We suggest using cast iron or stainless steel cookware.

Your drinking and cooking water is important to assess. Over one hundred chemicals have been identified in public drinking water, including antibiotics, other antimicrobials, estrogenic steroids, antidepressants, calcium channel blockers, chemotherapy drugs, and more. We suggest a point-of-use-activated carbon filter system or reverse osmosis for the home. One should be used on shower heads as well. Also, most plastic water bottles contain BPA, so switch to steel or glass. Test your well water annually for heavy metals and minerals.

Having the right kitchen appliances and gadgets will make

cooking and prep that much easier. Kitchen gadgets we suggest include,

• Food processor (for mixing, grating, slicing, and shredding)

• High-powered blender (such as a Vitamix or Ninja; basically a juicer that will keep the pulp for extra fibre and with which you can make nut milks, nut butters, and more)

• Dehydrator (great for making nut-and-seed granola and breads and drying surplus vegetables)

• Crock-Pot (makes cooking dinner a breeze; just throw ingredients in and by dinner soup is ready!)

• Recycling and compost setup (For the sake of our planet, please make space in your kitchen, garage, or storage area to sort glass, cans, plastic, and paper. Many cities will pick these items up for you. A small compost bins on the kitchen counter can be used to collect organic produce scraps, coffee grounds, organic teas, eggshells, and can enhance the nutrient density of the produce items you grow in your garden.)

Stocking Your Fridge, Freezer, and Pantry

When you hit the grocery store, the key is to stock up on fresh and frozen organic vegetables, low-sugar fruit, and fresh herbs. These foods should make up your diet's majority contents of your fridge. Ideally you will stock the fridge with cruciferous vegetables (like cabbage, broccoli, brussels sprouts), dark leafy greens (like collard, kale, spinach), onions (garlic, leeks, chives), and other vegetable families. Organic berries and green apples are great low-glycemic fruits. What's next on the list are organic, grass-fed meats, wild fish, pastured chicken and eggs, game meats, preservative-free shellfish, and nitrate-free organic bacon and sausage. Pre-prepared bone broths are great to have on hand and can be fresh or frozen.

Fermented foods and clean condiments (including sauerkraut; kimchi; pickles; gluten-free, sugar-free, preservative-free, and organic mustards, ketchup, salsas, and berry jams; coconut aminos; olives; Paleo mayo; horseradish; capers; and sun-dried tomatoes) are all great staples to have on board. Nuts, seeds, and their associated flours, milks, and oils should also be kept stocked. Extra nuts and seeds should be stored in glass jars in the freezer to preserve freshness. Pecans, walnuts, macadamia nuts, Brazil nuts, almonds, chia seeds, and flaxseeds are all great to have on hand. Olive, coconut, avocado, and MCT oils make fast, easy, and low-sugar salad dressings when combined with apple cider vinegar, chopped garlic, and herbs. Healthy beverages to keep stocked include sparkling water in glass containers, homemade iced green tea, kombucha, homemade kefir, and homemade nut milks with added herbs, such as turmeric.

In your pantry, stock canned full-fat coconut milk (without carrageenan), sustainably harvested tuna and sardines, sugar-free pasta sauce (glass jars are best), and olives. Dried herbs, mushrooms, spices, and teas are also important to have at home. The spice cabinet is the most healing part of the home. Dried teas, basil, oregano, turmeric, cumin, curry, coriander, bay leaves, thyme, rosemary, cinnamon, nutmeg, cayenne, tarragon, and others are the flavors you'll need! (Refill your bottles and buy in bulk to save money.) Crucial baking supplies include: baking soda, vanilla, cocoa nibs, nut flours, and shredded coconut. Sea vegetables include nori, wakame, arame, and seaweed snacks. These make great additions to soups. As you can see, there are so many low-glycemic and ketogenic-diet-friendly foods to bring into your house! So now that you are cleaned out and stocked with a nutrient-dense food supply, let's summarize the principles for following the most effective and potent anticancer diet ever developed.

SUMMARY OF PRINCIPLES OF THE METABOLIC APPROACH AND DIET

Within each chapter we have discussed many foods to incorporate into your diet and many to avoid. The key recommendation running through most of the chapters is to implement a low-glycemic, ketogenic-type diet that also incorporates intermittent fasting. There is so much therapeutic benefit obtained from not eating. But for starters, the number one secret to success when you change your diet is to focus on the foods you should be eating, not the ones that you should avoid. That mind-set will only set you up to feel deprived left out, and uninspired with your new diet. Rather, we want you to think of yourself as an ambassador for your health and an inspiration to others. You've learned about a powerful new therapy that can prevent or help manage cancer: food. Remember, there is no cancer diet which can fit everybody to lead an anticancer life. Each individual has a unique genetic code, a different cancer, and a different terrain. This is what makes our approach unparalleled.

There are three core principles to following this approach: low-glycemic; high-quality; and seasonal, diverse, and phytonutrient-dense foods. Since getting off sugar is a kind of coming off a drug, we spend some extra time on it in our three-tiered approach for those who need to take things step by step. So roll up your sleeves and get started. Here is what you need to focus on.

A TIERED APPROACH TO STARTING A LOW-GLYCEMIC DIET

The number one priority for this approach is to remove from your diet all sources of sugar and carbohydrates, aside from vegetables and low-sugar fruits. We always recommend following a ketogenic diet for those with active cancer to help halt the process. (Refer back to chapter 4 and chapter 5 for more details on diving into the ketogenic diet). Meanwhile, we have created a three-tiered process that leads comfortably toward the ketogenic diet. It doesn't matter which step you are ready to take first to decrease the intake of starch and sugar in your diet—every bite matters.

The first tier involves cutting the "whites"—white sugar and white flour (which should be a step adopted by everyone, no matter what).

The second tier involves removing gluten-containing grains because of the major negative impact they have on blood sugar, our genes, the immune system, inflammation, and mood balance. Not to mention that eating two pieces of whole wheat bread is equivalent to eating 2 tablespoons of sugar.

The third tier removes all grains, legumes, and other high-starch foods and replaces them with vegetables. This is the tier that gets people into a low-glycemic, plant-dense, therapeutic, and Paleo way of eating. This is a great place to land for those in remission, those with early-stage cancers, and those looking to prevent the occurrence of cancer. It's how Dr.Nasha and Jess advocate eating to everyone, and how they themselves eat. Look through these three tiers to determine which is the best starting point for you, or if you are ready to dive into the ketogenic diet.

TIER 1: KICKING THE WHITES

If you are just starting out with diet changes, have been eating a standard American diet, have a blood sugar disorder, or feel like you have low motivation and willpower for diet changes, then this is your zone. If removing things from your diet feels too restrictive, then we suggest first integrating the "crowd-out method" where you increasingly eat more vegetables (which will already make a positive impact on your terrain) while eliminating space for less healthy foods. You can revisit the sugar monster later, but always remember: Nothing is impossible. In this first tier, Jess has folks start out by tracking their sugar intake for three days—no diet change required. Read all labels and keep a running tally of how much sugar you eat and drink in a day. This includes sugar in your coffee and fruit.

Once you have a baseline for how much sugar you are eating, begin to decrease the amount by 10–20 percent every three to seven days. So if you are eating 150 grams of sugar a day, within seven days you want it down to 120 grams. Eventually, you want your sugar intake to be 20–40 grams a day or lower. By slowly decreasing the amount of sugar you may avoid the unpleasant effects of carbohydrate withdrawal, which can include fatigue, headaches, irritability, and other unpleasant symptoms. Once you get through the withdrawal period, which can last three weeks or more, you won't really miss sugar. Yes, really. We've heard it from patients over and over again. Your taste buds will change, and things that used to taste good will seem way too sweet to eat. Start by avoiding anything that contains white flour and white sugar (such as candy, cake, cookies, ice cream, and soda). Here are a few more tips for kicking the sugar habit:

Don't keep sugar-laden foods at home. Just like alcoholics cannot keep alcohol in the house, you cannot keep sugar in the house. The temptation is too great. Only keep enough for one serving. If guests bring sugar-rich foods over for a party, make sure they leave with them.

Remove corn from your diet. Since so much of the sugar in processed food comes from a corn base it's best to avoid corn as well. We've worked with people who are coming off sugar who report eating whole cans of corn, but were unsure where that craving came from. Chances are that if you've been eating a lot of sugar you are probably also allergic to corn.

Protein, protein, and more protein! Protein helps keep blood sugar levels stable thereby reducing cravings. Protein also helps to form the enzymes we need for digestion and gut healing as well as neurotransmitters such as serotonin. Eggs for breakfast are great, or—for those who are sensitive to eggs—do as they do in Eastern countries and have bone broth and kimchi for breakfast. If that sounds a little too extreme, think about meat and vegetables for breakfast, or a nut-and-seed granola.

TIER 2: REMOVE GLUTEN-CONTAINING GRAINS

After you feel like you are really on top of Tier 1 and ready to integrate more sugar-lowering changes into your diet, then you are ready for Tier 2. The important thing to remember here is that this is not a "diet" in the traditional sense of the word. You are making these changes forever, so you want to set yourself up for success, and for sustainability. Often people ask how long they have to stay gluten and sugar free. The answer is forever. So don't move on to Tier 2 until you feel like you are ready.

Now that you have learned how to look out for sugar, the next step is addressing the amount of carbohydrates in the form of grains in your diet, especially gluten-containing grains. Gluten-free diets are not fad diets, and consumption of modern wheat is incredibly destructive to our terrain, as you have discovered throughout this book.

- The Dos and Don'ts of a Gluten-Free Diet

Getting started can seem overwhelming. People will say, "But gluten is in everything!" We can assure you that gluten is not in everything, as evidenced earlier in the shopping in this chapter. For starters, take a grocery store tour. Many health food stores offer store tours where you can learn about (and sample!) many gluten-free foods. Next, it's important to start cooking. This is the centre piece to making diet changes. Learning how to cook will make it easier to follow the diet. Consider taking a cooking class or hiring a personal chef who can show you some basics. Then, calling on your awareness is important: Identify times of day, social situations, and specific comfort foods where you crave gluten-containing foods and replace those with new habits and routines. Reprogram.

Keep your mind-set away from deprivation and more toward abundance, health, and creativity. Communicate that you are gluten free because you want to be, not because you have to be. It's a healthy choice, much like exercising or eating organically. Let this be an opportunity for you to become an educator, not a victim, and welcome to an exciting new world of food! When you shop, read the labels on everything! Gluten can be found in many unexpected places (like in mustard, soy sauce, and processed meats). If you are unsure of an ingredient, contact the food manufacturer to confirm if a product you like is gluten-free or not.

Now for the don'ts, for newcomers to this approach, is that you should not skip meals. When blood sugar level starts dropping, cravings for high-carbohydrate foods will increase. Think about eating six small meals a day when starting out. Next, don't assume that because it's gluten-free it's healthy. There are many, many sugary, processed, GMO gluten-free foods out there. Finally, don't become overwhelmed or afraid of food. There are hundreds of things to eat that don't contain gluten. Fruits, vegetables, meats, fish, nuts, and seeds are all gluten free!

- Eating Out

For most people starting out with diet changes, knowing what to order when eating out can seem overwhelming, but don't despair. If all else fails, have a snack before eating out and enjoy some tea and a mini fast while enjoying the company of your friends and family. You don't have to eat to enjoy time with others, and connecting with other people as opposed to isolating yourself will help your terrain! The first step to eating out is getting to know what ingredients are likely to contain hidden gluten (many sauces, soy sauce, or anything that's breaded, for example) and not ordering those. We also suggest looking at the menu online ahead and calling the restaurant around 4 p.m. (if you are going out to dinner, that's before people have arrived and you're likely to get a manager who can confirm what can be made free of gluten).

Make sure to ask the waiter to check with the chef whether something contains gluten or how it is prepared. Speak to the manager before you order if it seems your waiter doesn't quite get it. Then, have confidence. It's hard, but try not to feel embarrassed or high-maintenance when requesting your food be gluten free. Your waiter doesn't have to sit in the chemo chair, you do. So speak up.

TIER 3: PALEO-TYPE, LOW-GLYCEMIC, AND NUTRIENT-DENSE

The jump from Tier 2 to Tier 3 means moving from a modern diet, to a diet more genetically in line with our ancestry and our genetics. It removes all foods that have been introduced since the advent of agriculture. This phase is where we really start to see therapeutic benefits—not just for cancer, but for all chronic illnesses. Here we take out all grains, both gluten containing and gluten free, as well as all beans (lentils, chickpeas, and black beans), all refined sugar, dairy, and all processed foods in general. This is a whole food, plant-based diet that includes quality proteins and healthy fats. This is the diet we try to get all our patients eating and then move to a ketogenic diet if they don't completely respond here.

This phase is very rich in vegetables. In fact, we recommend at least ten different types of vegetables every day, including at least two dark leafy greens vegetables, two cruciferous vegetables, two servings of garlic, onions, or shallots, two servings of mushrooms, one fermented vegetable, and one other that can include dark berries, eggplant, artichoke, bell peppers, asparagus, tomatoes, and so forth. The key thing to note about Tier 3 is that the only form of carbohydrate comes from vegetables or low-glycemic fruit, such as berries, bitter melon, and green apples.

This phase of the diet is also very high in fiber. Most people will lose weight on this diet. While this may alarm family members, you now know that there is a big difference between dangerous metabolic weight loss (cachexia) and therapeutic weight loss. There are some phenomenal cookbooks out there that can help get you started, including the 21-Day Sugar Detox, by Diane Sanfilippo, and Good Morning Paleo, by Jane Barthelemy. There are lots of tricks and tips for getting started on a Paleo-type diet. First off, the key is to get creative with vegetables: Cauliflower makes great rice; spaghetti squash and zucchini make amazing noodles. Vegetables should be the main event. Salad is the base for proteins. Dip artichoke leaves in a meat and liver sauce. And speaking of sauce that is where the secret is. Fish and vegetables can seem plain after a while, but zesting things up with a dill sauce or a red wine mushroom sauce makes dishes come to life. We encourage people to think about different cuisines, such as tacos on a cabbage leaf, lasagna layered with summer squash, or an Asian stir-fry with sprouts. It's also worth noting that having ethnic variety adds diverse flavor profiles to your dishes to prevent burnout.

Start going to farmers' market and grow your own vegetables to get the fresh and most flavorful and most nutrient-dense varieties. When children grow their own vegetables they are much more likely to eat them, not to mention it's a wonderful outdoor family activity. Next, if you are not following an autoimmune diet, try cooking with nut flours. You can make muffins, breads, pancakes, and all sorts of baked goods using almond, hazelnut, chestnut, sunflower, and coconut flours. Nuts and seeds also make great crusts for fish and chicken dishes. When making nut- or seed-flour baked goods, experiment with natural, low-glycemic sweeteners such as fresh stevia leaf, monk fruit sweetener, chicory root, green applesauce, or local or manuka honey. Desserts are for special occasions like holidays and birthdays, and these sweeteners are low in sugar and full of taste, with even a bit of therapeutic benefit.

Once people spend some time here in Tier 3 land, making the switch to a ketogenic diet is often not so daunting. It involves paring down vegetables to get daily carbohydrate intake somewhere close to 20 grams or less, while increasing fats to close to 120 grams in some cases. (Refer back to chapter 4 for more information.)

When it comes to managing cancer, the most therapeutic diet is a ketogenic one. We have explained in just about every terrain chapter how a ketogenic diet acts to: lower blood sugar, improve immune function, decrease inflammation, decrease metastases, and reset circadian patterns. Our hope is that now you have the tools and motivation to get started.

- Focus on Food Quality

The second core principle to taking a metabolic approach to cancer is to start choosing organic, sustainably raised (biodynamic) plants, animals, and animal by-products. Yes, we know that making the switch to organic may seem expensive. Between 1985 and 2000 the price of fruits and vegetables and fish increased up to 50 percent, while sugars and sweets and soda decreased by 25 percent. It is horrifying how broccoli is more expensive than a Dr Pepper! Nevertheless, what we tell people is that it sometimes takes looking at your budget and asking yourself questions like, "Which is more important, medicinal foods or new clothes every month?" It can necessitate a review of your priorities (oddly, it is sometimes the best-off people who have a hard time spending more money on food). Just as a reference point, however, Jess spends more money per month on groceries than on her mortgage.

As we've discussed throughout this book, conventionally raised animals are too toxic to eat. They are fed hormones, antibiotics, and genetically modified diets that increase their content of inflammatory omega-6 fatty acids. Not the best choice. Looking for 100 percent pasture-raised and wild-caught animals, or hunting your own, is how we suggest finding animal products. Animal by-products such as eggs and raw cheeses (if dairy is a part of your program) should come from those same animals. (Remember that if your ferritin levels are high, you want to avoid red meat. Your bio-individualized diet might differ in many ways from someone else's. It depends on your particular genetics and lab studies.)

We know that eating vegetables and low-glycemic fruit helps prevent cancer. Over two hundred epidemiological studies have found a consistent association between the low consumption of fruits and vegetables and cancer. When key micro- and phytonutrients are not present in the diet, DNA repair and immune functioning are impaired. Yet we also know that exposure to the pesticides used in the growing of these plants causes cancer. In 2012, a statement was issued by the American Academy of Pediatrics, urging children to reduce exposure to pesticides because of increased risk acute lymphocytic leukemia, brain tumor, reduction in IQ, and abnormal behaviors associated with autism and attention-deficit/hyperactivity disorder.

However, despite the documented adverse health effects of pesticides, their use has increased almost 25 percent in recent decades. Our continual low-dose exposure to these toxins increases the risk of genetic mutations, depletes our immune functioning, causes inflammation, and elicits an oxidative stress response in the body. Choosing organic or bio-dynamically raised produce items could not be more critical when it comes to the cancer crisis.

- Seasonal, Diverse, phytonutrient-Dense, and Properly Prepared

Think about changing your diet with the seasons. This is beneficial from both a preventive and a re-harmonizing standpoint. Start by visiting your local farmers market to see what foods are abundant in your area. As the bumper sticker says, "Know your farmer, know your food." In summer think about focusing on fish, eggs, vegetables, and fruit. In fall, eat red meat (it's hunting season) and poultry, along with herbs and cruciferous vegetables that are still growing in the garden. Winter is ketogenic and fasting time. This can be challenging for many people during the holidays with the cravings for sweet foods, but eating sweets is the opposite of what we should be doing! We highly encourage you to start new family traditions that are not steeped in sugar. In spring, it's time for renewal, and focusing on bitter greens to support the body's purging of the fatty foods of the winter can also help detoxify the body.

You may have noticed that there were several foods that were mentioned in just about every chapter as having the most powerful terrain actions: onions, garlic, turmeric, wild fish, mushrooms, green tea, broccoli, parsley, and dark leafy greens. (Try to have these every day.) As you get into the groove of eating seasonally, know that the micro- and phytonutrient content of all these foods is higher when they are in season. Also, many benefits of these foods are negated if they are cooked to high temperatures. We never bake over 300°F and also never sauté using high heat.

Now we will summarize each chapter and provide a corresponding recipe for you so that you can start improving your terrain with the most powerful natural medicine there is: food. To create these recipes, we incorporated foods from other chapters to make incredibly powerful, phytonutrient-dense and ketogenic-friendly recipes. Enjoy!

NOTES:

- The above mentioned 4 weeks diet plan is according to Rapid weight loss for a month. If you are planning to continue ketogenic type for more than one month and lose weight in a moderate rate, you can follow the meal plan of second week and third week alternatively.5 following the above mentioned diet plan you can lose 20 to 30 lbs during 4 weeks or maybe even more depending upon your rate of metabolism. If you feel that fasting in 4th week is too much intense for you can go back to second week's diet plan. You will still lose weight but not as much as you can lose by fasting.

- The food which are allowed to eat in keto diet are based on the the nutritional facts. By involving the allowed foods in your diet you will have a right approach to the recipes in keto diet. Avoid all the sugary drinks!

RESOURCES:

CHAPTER 7
How ketogenic diet works against cancer?

Before you start a ketogenic diet on your own, we suggest that you to consult a professional and get monitored because there are many clinical conditions in which you cannot follow this diet. It also includes some side effects which you might experience for some time, so it's better to consult a person to find out the side effects of a ketogenic diet.

Reducing intake of sugar and high glycemic food is the most important dietary step which can help patients to prevent and manage their cancer. It is the crucial way to weaken the metabolism of cancer cells. A Keto diet is the most powerful therapy that exerts protective anticancer effects. The keto diet is not a treatment for cancer, it can only prevent cancer! You will discover that there are nine other Terrain factors that contribute to cancer process but the most powerful effect is caused by sugar level in our blood. Therefore, a metabolic diet approach is an important effective tool that benefits all the other train areas to keep them in balance. The **ketogenic diet** is emerging as a stand-alone treatment for cancer being superior to all the Western medicines that has to offer for many cancer include in brain cancer, and is also a beneficial treatment of neurological condition such as epilepsy and Alzheimer's and Parkinson's disease. This is the reason why we refer ketogenic diet and fasting over and over again. Fasting and calorie restriction are not a new therapy, this has been practiced by people since the beginning of time when there were no therapeutic approach towards curing diseases.

In ancient times when there was scarcity of food people have experienced prolonged hours of hunger. Being hungry and going without food for long hours is known as fasting which was very common at that time. But, nowadays being hungry is a very uncomfortable feeling for many Americans. When was the last time you get yourself hungry for more than an hour? You might not remember this because as soon as you feel hungry, you snack on something like- chocolates nuts fruits berries on baked goods. The easy available processed foods contain a large amount of carbohydrates and sugar. Mostly baked goods like cakes, biscuits or cookies are packed and are easily available. So, whenever you feel hungry, instead of going and cutting fruits or making green tea, you just open a pack of baked goods and feed on it. They contain a large amount of calories because of sugar and carbs which ultimately harms our system.

How **ketosis** ultimately works is this: when body is deprived of dietary carbohydrates, the liver becomes the sole provider of stored glucose in the form of glycogen which it used to feed hungry organs like the brain. Brain is the organ which consumes most of the energy. It utilise this over 20% of the total energy produced by our body. Your liver stores only enough glucose to last the body somewhere between 24 to 48 hours. If humans didn't have a backup energy source, we would have extinct a long time ago. **Ketones** are power backup source of energy when our body lacks glucose. It works in the following way:

- Once the liver is depleted of glycogen- it starts making Ketone bodies either from fatty acid in the diet or from body fat. These ketone bodies are then released into bloodstreams which are taken up by the cells in the brain and other organs.
- These Ketone molecules are shuttled into mitochondria as energy factories just like glucose and are used to create ATP.
- Healthy cells have the ability to switch from utilising glucose (as energy fuel) to ketones. We have been

doing this since birth.
- Initial research has suggested that cancer cells lack this metabolic flexibility of switching from glucose to ketone and stops proliferating.
- The presence of ketone bodies lowers the levels of inflammatory cytokines. When ketones are used for energy in place of glucose or fatty acids, normal cells produce fewer ROS. Cancer cells, however, have defects in their mitochondria that don't allow them to efficiently use the ketogenic pathway. Many cancer cells also produce less of the specific enzyme needed to utilize ketones for energy, further increasing their vulnerability to metabolic stress.

The elimination of glucose from our blood is a state of nutritional ketosis which effectively Cuts of Cancer cells' main fuel supply and put them in a state of metabolic stress. Ketosis also provides other anticancer benefits including:

• Reduction in angiogenesis (formation of new blood vessels which supply fuel to the tumor cells)

• Restoring normal apoptosis in cancer cells (cell suicide process)

• Destabilizing tumor tissue DNA which causes effects that damage the cancer cells

• Gradual reduction in tumor size

• Insulin and IGF-1 levels reduction

• Enhancing the action of standard treatments, including chemotherapy and radiation, while reducing common side effects

It is true and has been proved by many researchers that sugar can make or break the conventional cancer treatment. It is a myth that ketogenic diet only helps brain cancer. All the cancer, except prostate broncho-alveolar lung cancer, mucinous adenoma of colon and thyroid cancer are highly glucose dependent.

Are you starting a ketogenic diet to prevent cancer? Know this:

Without specific nutrition, which is designed to repair mitochondrial dysfunction, invigorate the immune system and reduces inflammation resulting in imbalance of hormones and blood sugar forcing healthy cells to become uncontrollable and enter into realm of cancer. You might be wondering- how to achieve ketosis and start using ketones as a fuel opposed to glucose?

According to ketogenic diet, the general portions of an individual's daily nutrient intake for ketosis to work out is approximately- 70–75 percent of calories from healthy anti-inflammatory fats, 20–25 percent from quality proteins, and 5–10 percent from carbohydrates, which should consist of low-carbohydrate, phytonutrient-dense vegetables. The Atkins diet promoted high protein and moderate fat. Why does the ketogenic diet suggest instead a high-fat, moderate-protein ratio? It is because fats have no effect on blood sugar and insulin level protein can however affect both of these if consumed in large quantity. If too much of protein is consumed, then more than 50% of any excess protein will be converted into glucose, and that extra glucose can increase insulin level hampering the ketosis process in our body. Calorie intake and macronutrient ratios need to be assessed and reassessed on an individual basis. However here is an approximate example of what a 2000 calorie per day diet should look like:

- Fat (9 calories per gram) = 165 grams or 1,500 calories
- Protein (4 calories per gram) = 100 grams or 400 calories
- Carbohydrate (4 calories per gram) = 25 grams or 100

calories

Carbohydrates have the biggest impact on glucose level that is why they are consumed in smallest amount in keto diet and should come from the most nutrient dense and low glycemic vegetable this includes dark green fresh herb, mushroom, garlic and onion. A legitimate criticism of the ketogenic diet is its low amount of phytonutrient rich vegetables. It is possible to eat a good amount of lemon, lime, basil, broccoli, cilantro, spinach, garlic and more everyday and still remain in ketosis. The main goal will always remain to infuse most nutrient dense food into ketogenic diet plan. Every individual's response towards ketogenic diet is different: some achieve ketosis with a larger amount of carbohydrate intake- like 30 grams or more; while other must lower their carbohydrate diet intake below 20 gram to start ketosis. Some people can achieve a 10 vegetable a day gold diet while following ketogenic diet. When you first start your diet the most important thing is- to have a track record of your carbohydrate intake. Always, try to keep it below 20 grams a day.

Since healthy anti inflammatory fats and quality protein contributes towards the majority portion of ketogenic diet, let's take a closer look at their benefits:

- **Healthy fats and oils:**

Saturated and monounsaturated fats are healthier over unsaturated fatty acids. You should avoid hydrogenated fats to reduce trans-fat intake. Use "cold pressed" organic brand's vegetable oils. Almond and flaxseed oil are "cold pressed", and should be kept refrigerated to limit rancidity. Use coconut oil, olive oil and ghee for frying, since they have high smoke points and are non-hydrogenated. Try to avoid heating vegetable oils.

- Beef tallow
- Ghee is butter with milk solids removed

- Almond oil.
- Avocado oil
- Butter
- Non hydrogenated lard
- Avocado
- Organic chicken or duck fat
- Macadamia nuts.
- Mayonnaise, no or low sugar.
- Macadamia oil.
- Organic olive oil
- Coconut oil, coconut butter and coconut cream concentrate (all should be organic)
- Red palm oil (organic)
- Olives, green and black.
- 90 % dark chocolate in very small amounts
- Unsweetened peanut butter.
- Oil of most seeds and nuts

DAIRY FATS

Following are listed sources of fats from dairy products. Try to get organic sources which are generally healthier overall.

- Butter.
- Sour cream (full fat)
- Ghee
- Organic cream cheese
- Mascarpone cheese
- Heavy whipping cream
- Beverages (all unsweetened)

- **Quality Proteins:**

    1. Animal protein:

Animal proteins have low amount of carbohydrates so when it comes to selecting animal food quality is very important.
- Fresh shellfish such as shrimp lobsters and scallops
- Salmon, mackerel, halibut, cod, haddock and sardines.
- Organic Turkey
- Grass fed beef and lamb
- Organic raised chickens and their eggs

    2. Dairy Proteins

Clean and organic dairy foods are good sources of protein nutrition, but they should be generally avoided on the ketogenic diet because of the following reasons:

- Fermented milk items like - cheese and yogurt, they are low in lactose, but, are also rich in casein

(milk protein), and so it is better to minimize their intake.
- Milk contains lactose (milk sugar) and casein- both increase insulin levels.
- Milk-based whey protein powders should be limited. Rice, hemp and vegetable protein powders are generally tolerable.

TESTING FOR KETOSIS:

When you are on keto diet to starve cancer cells, it becomes very important to often check your ketosis process. You should have a watch on how your body is responding towards ketosis. The presence and amount of ketones can be known either by using urine blood for the breath. Most of the people find that urine test strips are the easiest and most affordable home testing option; however, blood and breadth tests are slightly more accurate. Your body is said to be technically in ketosis when the blood Ketone levels reach a level of 0.5mmol/L. for individuals with active cancer Ketone levels are generally kept at or above 3.0mmol/L and glucose levels at 70mmol/L or lower. There are home testing options that can read both ketones and glucose levels in the blood. One of them is precision extra blood glucose monitoring system and another tool used in clinical setting is the glucose Ketone index calculator which is designed by Dr. Thomas Seyfried, which monitors therapeutic levels of ketone.

NOTES:

- By reading this chapter you will come to know about the food we eat gets metabolized to produce energy and assist in the building of protein to make immune cells, DNA and so forth. When fewer calories are consumed the amount of nutrients available to the body's cell is lowered. This in turns lowers metabolic process, reduces the production of free radical, and limits the function and expression of some protein involved in the cancer process. You can look up for cancer cells metabolism in other chapters and that how it depends upon glucose to proliferate.

REFERENCE:

CHAPTER 8

Is keto diet always beneficial?
Benefits of keto diet

- Low cholesterol levels.

It is made from extra amount of glucose in your body which is not used for energy production, so when we eat less amount of carbohydrate our cholesterol level drops and HDL level increases as we consume more saturated fat, which is a good thing. Triglyceride level decreases because they are closely related to the amount of carbohydrate you consume.

- Lack of Hunger.

Beneficial fats are very satisfying, as they break down to form ketone bodies which suppress hunger. It may make you forget about eating by decreasing your starvation and craving for food.

- Less stiffness and joint pain.

A fact says that grain-based foods increase inflammation and causes many chronic diseases especially in overweight people.

- Lower blood sugar and insulin levels.

Insulin hormone is released as a response of sugar in our blood stream. Lower the sugar level floating in bloodstream lower will be the level of production of insulin.

- Reduced fogginess.

The brain is made up of at least 50% facts by weight so the more you each fat the more your brain can maintain itself.

- Increased energy.

At the start of keto diet you will experience some muscle fatigue, but once you get adapted to it, your energy level will increase a lot.

- Constant sleep pattern.

Sleep apnea is generally caused due to high carb consumption which can cause heartburn. You will no longer require an afternoon nap that generally disrupts your circadian rhythm.

- Weight loss.

As your energy source dependence changes, you will start losing some weight, provided you become healthy in this process. After an initial Rapid weight loss, you might feel that you have stopped losing any further weight; this condition is a diet plateau (where you stop losing weight). By combining a routine exercise with your diet you can lose more weight while building toned muscles without feeling hungry.

- Relief from gastric symptoms.

The high carb diets are the main cause of heartburn, improper digestion and GERD. Symptoms will slowly disappear when you follow ketogenic diet. If you still experience heartburn consult to your physician to examine gallbladder function and eliminate tomatoes from your diet. The lower intake of grains-based and sugars-based foods eliminate the process of fermentation in your small intestine; hence, you will be relived from gas and bloating.

- Increase in dopamine and serotonin levels.

Ketone bodies can calm down body's neurotransmitter, and results in fever mood swings which allow you to feel happy in general. It is the time when a person taking selective serotonin reuptake inhibitors can know that - whether, he should continue taking those medications, or if, he can remove that medicine from his routine.

- Oral health improvement

Sugar causes tooth decay by changing the pH of mouth. After 2-3 months of keto diet you will feel that any kind of oral problem you were experiencing has disappeared.

Side effects of keto diet

- Fatigue, dizziness muscle cramp and headache.

In keto diet we lose a considerable amount of electrolytes like sodium, potassium and magnesium which causes the feeling of fatigue and dizziness. Consuming sea salt in your food can help you to replace those minerals which are lost.

- Frequent urination.

For every gram of glycogen, 324 gram of water is also stored in your muscles, so when the body starts to burn glycogen-- your kidney begins to get rid of excess of water stored.

- Constipation.

It is usually very common to have constipation while being on ketogenic diet. It dehydrates your body and cause the loss of a considerable amount of salt. Eating too many nuts or having a magnesium imbalance in body can also be the reason of constipation.

- Hypoglycaemia.

It is a condition where blood sugar level drops down. Your body was used to produce a certain amount of insulin when you were consuming foods loaded with carbohydrates. As your carbohydrate intake is reduced, you might experience low blood sugar level for sometime before your body totally adapts to new metabolism.

- Diarrhoea.

It is usual to have diarrhoea in the beginning which will be settled after a few days even without taking medicines, but, you can have self medication by taking a spoon of sugar free Metamucil or an anti-diarrheal just before your meals until diarrhoea stops to occur.

- Kidney stones.

This is a very rare side effect. Before taking any potassium citrate supplement you should consult to your physician- if you have kidney for blood pressure problem.

- Sleep changes.

You might experience change in sleep pattern due to decreased serotonin or insulin levels; and this may be an indication that you are unable to tolerate high amount of histamine. This effect varies from person to person. If you find difficulty in sleeping you can have some snacks just before going to bed which should contain protein with a little amount of carbohydrate in it.

- Sugar cravings

This can last for 2 to 3 weeks where you can experience intense sugar cravings. The lasting effect of sugar craving depends on how much carbohydrate you have consumed. You can overcome this feeling by consuming protein. Try to distract your mind whenever you crave for sugar.

- Low T3 thyroid hormone levels

When our body gets into ketosis, it becomes susceptible to T3 thyroid hormone levels; therefore, you do not require it as much. It's more a natural consequence of getting into keto diet than a side effect!

- Heart palpitations

There are several reasons for this side effect which are
  1. Lowest blood pressure

2. Transient hypoglycaemia
3. Electrolyte imbalance or dehydration
4. Too much consumption of MCT oil such as coconut oil
5. Less intake of protein

- Hair loss

This may occur due to imbalance of insulin level. Once your body insulin level comes to normal the hair loss will stop and it will be fuller as it becomes healthier.

The above mentioned side effects last only for a small period of time because our body requires time to get adjust to new metabolism. Ketogenic diet built up our muscle and immune system. It also has a therapeutic use as it stars cancer cells, so ketogenic diet is really worthy to build up a Healthy body and lifestyle.

Is ketogenic diet dangerous? Find out that it's a myth or truth?

You might have heard that ketogenic diet is dangerous because it contains high amount of fats which can lead to heart related diseases. This is just a myth passed on by people who are less aware of the body metabolism related to digestion of carbohydrates and fats. Though there might be some side effects which remain for a short period of time; there are enormous benefits of having ketogenic diet.

- Eating fat will make you fat is the biggest myth you will ever hear. This has been taught to us since ever, without any scientific proof or fact. Actually, the fact is that - a diet containing high amount of carbohydrate will increase your sugar and insulin levels in your bloodstream, which can cause inflammation in your body. The fats you eat in ketogenic diet are healthy for your body because they are saturated fats (which are healthy). American studies have shown that a combination of saturated fatty acids with high carbohydrate diet is the reason for heart disease. Ketogenic diet contains very low carbohydrates and high amount of saturated fat that results in reduction in inflammation because of reduced glucose and insulin levels in your blood.

- The second criticism says that - saturated fats and cholesterol, if consumed in high amount, will cause heart diseases. This line has been passed on to one another since multiple decades. Johns Hopkins medical school had a study on low carb diet, and suggests that ketogenic diet is healthy because it contains high amount of saturated fats. Highest saturated fat increases high density cholesterol which is also called good cholesterol; while low carbohydrate intake decreases triglyceride levels (both are responsible for heart disease). Studies have shown that heart diseases are caused by taking high carbohydrate diet on a daily basis and not by eating saturated fat.

- Third criticism is that the keto diet does not give proper result to some people. This is absolutely false! As we have suggested in this book that you should seek advice from your doctor before starting this diet plan to know that you are medically fit for it or not! There are certain medical conditions in which you should avoid following ketogenic diet all be strictly supervised by your medical care provider.

- The forth criticism is likely to occur- that is- the person following this diet may have some chances to fall into the risk of ketoacidosis. It is not just caused by keeping your die body into ketosis. It occurs when there is unusually high amount of ketone bodies in the blood brought on by an irregulated metabolic reaction. ketoacidosis normally occur in individuals having Type 1 Diabetes (people who cannot produce insulin of their own). Nutritional ketosis is a self regulated process which allows enough insulin to remain in the blood to balance the level of ketones, preventing ketoacidosis. The only way some people following ketogenic diet might develop ketoacidosis are:

1. If a person is in starves for some months. Ketoacidosis does not occur with the suitably planned meal.
2. If a person performs high intensity exercise for prolonged period.
3. If a person is chronic alcoholic who indulge in extreme drinking

KETOACIDOSIS (ITS EFFECTS):

Some medical researchers and doctors gets confuse between diabetic ketoacidosis and benign nutritional ketosis. Diabetic ketoacidosis is an extreme and dangerous form of ketosis, while the benign nutritional ketosis linked with ketogenic diets and fasting. As you know that insulin regulates ketone production, so the difference between the two type of ketoacidosis is dependent upon the condition that, whether the body has the ability to make insulin or not!

- Benign nutritional ketosis is regulated by insulin, which results in a mild liberation of fatty acids and conversion of a fair amount of fatty acids into ketone bodies.
- Diabetic ketoacidosis a condition in which insulin is absent, either because the pancreas cannot produce it (Type 1 Diabetes) or body cells are insulin resistant (Type 2 Diabetes). Therefore, blood glucose level increases and unwanted amount of ketones are produced in an unregulated biochemical process.

Ketoacidosis is dangerous because ketone bodies are produced in the amount. In the absence of insulin a large amount of it is produced at once, so they build up in the bloodstream. The total volume quickly affects the weak acid-base buffering system of the blood. Since the ketone bodies are slightly acidic in nature, they make blood more acidic than normal. This condition of blood becoming more acidic is dangerous in case of ketoacidosis and not the ketones themselves.

- Following are list of profits coupled with a ketogenic diet.

1. Decreased Blood Pressure: diets containing low amount of

carbs are very helpful in decreasing blood pressure. Blood pressure medications cause the feeling of dizziness because of too much medication so before taking it, make sure that you are aware of the consequences. You should talk to your doctor about reducing blood pressure medication.

2. Better Heart Health: higher intake of saturated fat increases the amount of HDL. Increasing of HDL is actually a good for us, because it increases the ratio of HDL/LDL. A higher HDL level (above 39 mg/dL) gives an indication of a healthy heart.

3. Reduced Triglyceride level: Triglyceride in blood is a sole indicator of heart disease risk and the level of it is related to the amount of carbohydrate consumption. If you are suffering from conditions such as insulin resistance or metabolic syndrome, then eating less carbohydrate can effectively lower down your triglyceride readings.

4. Lower Average Blood Glucose level: Your fasting and after meal blood sugars will gradually drop, as you start eating low carbohydrate food. An average of your blood glucose levels can be seen on a haemoglobin A1C test, which is a long term measure of average blood glucose and takes up to 3 months. Since a ketogenic diet results in lowering of blood sugar level, this amount should decrease over time.

5. Lowers down Insulin Levels: Lowering down of blood sugar marks in lowering of insulin level. It is the most important payback of a keto diet, as it is related to many other health related factors such as inflammatory markers and IGF-1 levels.

6. Lowers down Level of Inflammation: The keto diet results in reduction of blood glucose and insulin levels, so it is an inflammatory diet. The levels of these two in blood are most influential inflammatory triggers and they are mostly stimulated by nutritional preferences. Inflammation level in body can be calculated by using a test called "C Reactive Protein test", or CRP in short. It calculates the inflammation of whole body, and also indicates the risk of heart disease. The CRP level drops when

you start a keto diet because your blood insulin and glucose drop.

7. Increase in energy levels: Energy will increase to a considerable amount as the body will burns fat for fuel instead of glucose. Each gram of fat contains double the amount of calories than each gram of glucose, therefore, when each gram of fat is burnt, it gives more energy than glucose. You will also be somewhat relieved from any chronic fatigue symptoms you might be having.

8. Reduced Joint pain and stiffness: Carbohydrate foods are the main cause of chronic illness and pain, particularly muscle stiffness and joint pain and keto diet help in eliminating carbs from our daily diet. The agenda of no grain, no pain is applicable here!

9. Clear mind: A high carb diet also causes brain "fogginess", it will start to disappear while you are on keto diet. The brain made up of 60% of fat by weight, I believe that the more fat you eat, the better your brain can maintain itself for working to its full capacity. Reduction of fogginess may also help in lowering inflammation in brain.

10. Decrease in unwanted Hunger: Fat gives the sensation of fullness for a longer time as it requires more time to digest than carbs do! And ketone bodies have proven to suppress appetite. You might forget to eat regularly, as you will not be dealing with small cravings. This is the most amazing part of keto diet, especially if you are addicted to food.

11. Heartburn Relief: Symptoms of problems like GERD or other heartburn problems can be lessen or vanish when you follow keto diet. Eating carb based foods, sugar and for some people nightshade vegetables like bell peppers can also be the reason of heartburn. Keto diets do not permit these categories of foods.

12. Reduces Tooth and gum problems: Carbohydrates results in tooth decay by changing its pH of your mouth which results in decaying of tooth. Following ketogenic diet for 3 months, you

will feel that your mouth has becomes much healthier.

13. Improved Digestion power: Digestive problems like stomach pain, gas, bloating will disappear after being on the keto diet for several days. These problems are linked with sugar and grain-based food intake.

14. Stabilized frame of mind: Studies have proven keto diet to be very effective in healing of mind health problems such as Schizophrenia and Depression.

15. Stressing the factors linked with Cancer: A keto diet will cause a drop in levels of sugar, insulin and insulin-like growth factor 1 (IGF-1) in blood, which can put metabolic stress on cancer cells and decline their development rate.

NOTES:

Nutritional ketosis is not dangerous, because keto diet is formulated properly with a balance of right meal plans and moderate exercises. Ketosis is a normal metabolic process that is completely safe for a person who is not suffering from diabetes. A person who is a severe alcoholic might have the risk of ketoacidosis.

REFERENCE:

https://www.diabetes.co.uk/blood-glucose/ketosis.html

https://www.healthline.com/nutrition/ketosis-safety-and-side-effects

CHAPTER 9

How does ketogenic diet works for losing weight?

When you eat a diet saturated with carbohydrates, it is broken down into glucose in your body. This glucose is stored in the form of glycogen in your liver that is broken up into simple glucose whenever the need for energy arises in the body. Insulin is created by your pancreas for converting glycogen to glucose, so it can be absorbed in your bloodstream and move around in your body.

When glucose is being utilized for fuelling your body, the fats in your body are just lying around in the form of bulky tissues. They aren't used because your body is relying on glucose for providing it with the necessary strength and energy to keep going. This problem results in weight gain and paves the way for obesity. It is this fatty issue that the ketogenic diet targets.

When you start a ketogenic diet, you switch to foods that are rich in fats instead of carbohydrates. As you take less carbohydrate, your body gets a smaller supply of glucose to be used for energy as compared to before. The decrease in the consumption and supply of carbohydrates forces your body to slowly move into ketosis.

If, this is your first encounter with the logic of eating fat to lose fat, you might probably be wondering- how this works? Well, for starters, when you take food, which is high in fat, your body starts breaking it down for energy, a process, which ends up producing adenosine triphosphate or simply ATP. Ketones are a product of the process. So when you ingest less carbs, you push the body to start burning more fat and in the process, you end up producing more ketones some of which are very important for energy production like ß-hydroxybutyrate and acetoacetate. It is perhaps important to know that your heart and the kidneys prefer ketones to glucose. Additionally, the brain cells can also use ketones for energy. However, acetone, which is one of the types of ketone molecules produced is not used for energy and is instead released as waste through urine and breath. So the more ketones you produce, the more of acetone you pass through urine. You can test acetone levels in your urine using a dipstick. This is how you can test if you're in a state of ketosis or not – you only get into a state of ketosis if your ketones are high enough to be detected in these tests.

When you go on a ketogenic diet, your goal is to get your body into a glycogen deprived state then stay in this state for some time as you maintain what is known as mild state of ketosis (in this case, you are converting fat into energy).

If there is a mild state of ketosis, this means that there is an optimal state, right? So how can you achieve a state of optimal ketosis where you are running on fat and your insulin level is at its lowest? Well, the secret is in avoiding all sources of carbs then take more proteins (of course in moderation). Your goal is to provide just enough proteins to make sure that the body is not forced to burn muscle tissue for energy because this might end up causing muscle loss and even increase insulin levels- some of the protein is converted to glucose. If you keep the protein levels sufficient, fats high, and carbs to almost zero, you will end up burning most fat and ultimately achieve optimal ketosis. This might take anywhere between 2-7 days depending on your activity level, what you eat and your body type.

You should also note that the body takes time to adapt to using ketones and fats as a source of energy. That's why you might experience some of negative effects at first like weakness, mild irritability, fatigue, or light headedness. However, this should be gone after your body adjusts, typically within a week.

Moderate exercise for weight loss:

Despite the many physical and emotional benefits of regular exercise, you may not feel like you can begin or maintain a regular routine. However, once you are keto-adapted, you may find that you feel better and have more energy than expected. The metabolic changes that accompany the shift to ketosis can improve your well-being even as you move through treatment. This improved quality of life is one of the surprising and very desirable side effects of anticancer ketogenic metabolic therapy.

What should you do if you stop losing weight on a keto diet?

In all diet most people reach a state where they stop losing weight. This state is called a **diet plateau**, where we continue the same habits but cannot lose weight. For some people, it might occur after 6 months of starting a diet but for some it might approach after a year all to of dieting. This plateau can last anywhere from a few days to 2-3 months. You require both motivation and special strategies to break through this period.

Some people might assume that they have reached a plateau only after a couple weeks of dieting but it actually isn't a plateau it is the water weight that they lose. As you start keto diet your body begins to use up all it stored sugar which releases water on breakdown. This water loss leads to a false sense of weight loss.

Cause of Plateau:

- Hidden carbs-
Carbs are practically present in almost all foods from baked goods grains and cereals to keto friendly foods like fruits and vegetables. Carbohydrates are often hard to

avoid because they are the important part of every food. But, on Keto diet it is important to know the amount of carbohydrate you are consuming to keep you in ketosis. Hidden cards can be found out by knowing the ingredients of your food. If, you need more information on understanding the nutrition labels check the comprehensive keto diet nutritional charts for more details.

- Keto fat bombs-

Like any other diet keto diet also has some treats and junk foods to hit those macros. Keto treats are very high in fat so consuming a lot of them can lead to plateau. Even though fat is allowed in higher amount for kid's diet, consumer eats more than what is needed which leads to storage of the extra fats. Keep your fat intake in a moderate level as per the calculation planned in your meal plan.

- Confusing macros-

You might often get confused between percentage skill and gram scale. The portion chart as mentioned in previous chapter contains carbs in grams protein in lbs and fat in percentage. We recommend you to stick to one measurement scale to keep track of your food using only that. Tracking your macros and calories is very beneficial for you until you are able to recognise your portion size.

Overcoming plateau:

There are following 15 ways to overcome plateau-

- Cut down carbohydrate intake.

You might be unknowingly taking more amount of carbohydrates as per suggested in the portion of heater diet. Search for the nutritional label of every food you eat to keep account it on the daily carbohydrates intake.

- Cut down on fats.

Although, fat is allowed in high amount in a keto diet, but

you should take only that much amount of fat which your body can burn. It depends upon your rate of metabolism and the rate of your physical activity. If you do a lot of exercise everyday you can take high amount of fats but if you are a lazy person you should cut down your intake of fat.

- Include more fibre in your diet.

Fibre contains no carbohydrates, proteins, or fats. They are the indigestible part of the food which absorbs and retains water, helping us to feel full between two meals while keeping us away from unnecessary craving of snacks.

- Switch to green tea.

Switch to green tea from tea or coffee, as it contains phenols which acts as antioxidants and these antioxidants increases your rate of metabolism which interns fastens the fat burning process.

- Increase intensity of exercise.

Your metabolic rate slows down if you don't keep yourself active. The amount of fat you have been taking which should be utilised for energy making gets stored in the body if you don't utilise it. Practice high intensity interval training (HIIT) in every two to three days a week including aerobics and weight lifting

- Have a cheat meal.

When you lose weight you also lose fat less fat results in less production of leptin which is a satiety hormone. Low amount of leptin hormone tells the brain to conserve calorie to prevent starving. You can feed on a cheat meal to regain the process of leptin production to restart weight loss process.

- Cut down on salt.

Sometimes you don't seem to lose weight because of water retention in your body. This can be caused due to number of reasons but the most common cause of this is too much consumption of sodium filled processed food. We never excrete sodium ions in urine- so, to keep a moderate level of sodium ions in our blood and cells water returns in our body to maintain osmoregulation. The more amount of salt you consume the more water will be written test in your body cells.

- Drink more water before meals.

Drinking more water 15 to 30 minutes before meals gives you the senses of fullness and prevents you from eating much.

- Increase your protein intake.

Navigate the amount of protein you are consuming and increase its portion. Eating good quality and organic protein is very important.

- Vary your workout.

Mix your workout pattern and try a new activity of sport like tennis, boxing, or swimming. When, you have a regular workout routine your muscle becomes familiar with the same exercise regularly and your mind attached to it. Our body is very smart it learns how to do all that exercises using few calories, which is the reason for or seizing of further weight loss.

- Note down your daily food intake.

Make a journal of things you eat everyday and calculate the calorie content in it. At the end of the day, you will be able to know the amount of calories you are taking. In this way you will be able to know that, are you consuming more than what is required. Research shows that people who note down their daily progress are more successful in weight loss

- Get quality sleep.

Late night sleep kills your weight loss progress! Lack of

sleep can make you feel groggy and a prolonged experience of it can cause long term side effects and change your metabolism for the worse. If our brain does not get enough quality sleep it stresses out and imbalances the entire hormone levels which affects our metabolism. Buy quality sleep I mean those 6 to 8 hours of sleep **at night.**

- Take a rest day.

If you are doing high intensity interval exercise (HIIT), take 1 to 2 days of rest in between those days. You use your mobile for almost 10 hours a day, and keep it at rest for charging it during overnight, or at any time of the day when it fully discharges. In the same way your body also needs rest after HIIT to recharge itself. Giving your mind the appropriate time to regain its ability of intensely working out will put you back on the track of your weight loss journey. Taking a few days off from gym is also a reward of overtraining.

- Always be active.

Hitting the gym for one or two hours a day and lying on the couch for the rest of the day will not do any good for your weight loss. Always try to keep you moving rather than sitting in one place for a long period. Resting your body is different from being lazy. A nap in the daytime is good but only after you have earned it by being active all day. Try to burn extra calories by doing some household works like cleaning your stuffs with hand without the help of any kind of machine.

- Always be motivated.

When you are in your plateau don't let yourself be demotivated. You can lose confidence and be off-track from your weight loss strategies if you think you cannot lose any further weight. Always keep your mind positive towards losing weight and stick to your proper diet plan. Find your mistakes you have been making by eating more amount of carbohydrate than suggested for remaining active throughout the day.

NOTES;

If you are diabetic, you should get advice from your physician first- before going on a keto diet because you might end up triggering what is known as diabetic ketoacidosis. When you are in this state, you have extremely (and potentially dangerous levels) of ketones in your body. However, if you are healthy, your ketosis is referred to as dietary ketosis, physiological ketosis, nutritional ketosis or benign dietary ketosis.

Reference:

https://theketokettle.com/keto-diet-plateau-how-to-break-through/

https://www.healthline.com/nutrition/weight-loss-plateau#section8

https://www.eatthis.com/weight-loss-plateau/

CHAPTER 10
Do you want to live a cancer free life? Follow the tips...

To cope up with your disease you have to make a considerable amount of change in your lifestyle. Side effects of treatment may leave you too tired to maintain your normal routine and you might have to change your work hours to accommodate your treatments schedule. There is loss of income on cancer treatments which deplete your savings and even put you to a temporary hold on your leisure but these unwelcome modifications are often a necessary part of the new norm: your cancer lifestyle. Your diagnosis can be a catalyst for positive Lifestyle changes so balance your new nom by developing your own unique anticancer life style. Here are few tips which can help cancer patient to live a positive and healthy life:

- **Reduce your stress level**

  Stress has a very great impact on immune system and overall metabolism and also has a direct impact on blood glucose level. Stress can make or Break your anti cancer life style so cultivate an awareness of your personal stress and live the life to the fullest.

- **Stay away from bad world news**

  We rely on media to stay connected to the world. But in recent years it has been filled with negativity and hatred. It is no longer a part of early morning routine which can start your day with something good. It can only fill your mind with negativity and stress. It's constant everywhere and has become more polarized over time. Limit your exposure to both online and from television news.

- **Recognize negativity**

Sometimes we all have negative thoughts and emotions overpower in our conscious mind. Move past them and let them go away so that they do not enter hijacking your day. Do mindfulness practices such as meditation, yoga or tai chi to calm down your mind and soul if you are stressed out with negative thoughts. These practices have shown to lower markers of inflammation. Create a countless variation between these exercises by balancing both restoring and energizing practices.

- **Don't overburden yourself**

Do you ever feel that you haven't done anything enough for the day? This question might come in your mind if you are expecting too much from yourself. Make a note of everything you do you in that day, it will help you to keep a a track on what you do and will give you a state of mindfulness when you look at all the work you did on that day. and keep a wave unrealistic expectations from yourself and always keep yourself motivated.

- **Detach from screen**

Getting too much exposed to electronic waves coming out of the screen from your Smartphone, laptop, tablet, TV and video games can pressurize your eyes and mind causing a headache and Visual impairment. Start cutting your exposure to screen by avoiding TV and tablet. Exposing yourself to mild sun rays is very beneficial for your skin in contrast to blue light emitted from devices like LED bulbs which is known to disrupt the circadian rhythm and sleep pattern.

- **Spend time in nature**

You cannot live life without nature, it is an integral part of our ecosystem and we are solely related to it for existence. Being close to natural world motivates you to lead a healthy life. Spend some time outdoor by walking or riding bicycle in parks of forest.

There are plenty of other activities to help you enjoy life and reduce your stress:

• Spend time socializing; we're hard-wired to connect!

• Listen to music, sing, or play an instrument.

• Watch a comedy or read a light-hearted book.

• Laugh a lot.

• Express your creative side through painting, pottery, crafts, and textile arts (among others).

• Volunteer!

• Travel for pleasure.

• Write, or keep a journal.

• Enjoy a spa day!

• Acknowledge a special person in your life who is a source of strength and support, then call or send the individual a text expressing your appreciation.

- **Get good sleep**

Good sleep is very important and Critical to health and well being. Very few people especially get good quality of sleep. Buy good quality of sleep I mean 8 hour of sleep at night without any disturbance. You should sleep in right posture and free your mind from any stress before sleeping.

There are so many health ailments related to deprivation of sleep like muscle factory stress on brain and eyes dark circles dizziness improper digestion etc. Don't use your mobile phone before bed as it causes sleep deprivation. Your mind and body needs rest at a particular time of day. After having in 8 hours sleep in the night you will wake up with a fresh mind and energetic body.

- **Do moderate exercise everyday**

Take out some time from your heavy schedule to practice moderate exercise. Although you have heavy skid use of treatments and other appointments make exercise your first priority in the morning. Here are some tips to keep you moving:

• Keep your walking shoes and water bottle near the front door.

• Bookmark your favorite yoga video, or leave a DVD near your TV.

• Store your yoga or exercise mat and light weights in an easy-to-access space.

You might start by only a 5 minutes' walk. But that's a great start! Keep it light at initial state

Set a goal to keep moving without getting exhausted.

How long should you remain on ketogenic diet?

This is a common question: "how long do I have to stay on this diet?" people have been asking this question very frequently. I want to tell them that you too jenny diet is much more than just a diet! There are so many benefits ghost to your body by this diet, it not only site steps diseases but also slowest down the agent of our body. You can surely liberal eyes your diet plan overtime using a glucose metre to test your body's response to specific food or meal. First week of starting this diet and most challenging and research says that it typically takes several months to develop news habit. Once you get keto adopted it will serve you for a lifetime

- **Fully commit to it for at least 12 weeks before changing it up:**

12 weeks is the time when majority of people see result of a diet. Once you are adapted to Keto you might play with your plan to see if little variations affect the glucose and Ketone number to significant amount. By this time you might have learn how to control yourself and stay away from common foot traps containing hidden carbs and sugar that may have kicked you out of ketosis.

Adopting a new way of thinking about food as nutrition rather than food as comfort will make your mind set change for better choices of food and you will be able to take more informed decisions regarding what to eat it as you continue on your journey. You can have some non key to food during keto holidays, but have a periodical test to be sure that you are Ketone levels are staying above the threshold for nutritional ketosis (0.5 mmol/L), indicating that you are still using fats and ketones as a source of energy.

- **Keep in mind**

You should always have some basic points to Remember like-

- Eat only small portions of berries and certain low-glycemic fruits.

- Keep protein portions low but adequate to meet your needs.

- Limit dairy proteins portions.

- Don't forget to include lots of healthy fats and oils!

- **Long term lifestyle in keto diet**

If you are practicing keto diet on a life long term basis you no need to fast in the fourth week as per suggested in the plan. You can follow thousand of keto recipes available in many e books and sites. I will suggest you some books (just click the link down below) for many recipes. Whenever you go outside pack your own snacks and food to avoid the high carb meals available in the market. Does it seem a little hard work to do you but 800000 and be achieved without doing anything for yourself? Once you get adapted to keto life you will have a great power of avoiding all the unhealthy foods.

- **Navigate sick days**

Glucose and Ketone levels can fluctuate when you are ill or injured. Therefore, whenever you are sick test your glucose and Ketone levels. If, any complication occurs you should seek medical care.

Nausea and vomiting are usual side effects in people who are getting conventional cancer treatment. If, you want to eat on chemo therapy days you may feel more comfortable if you take fewer amounts of fats more amounts of proteins and divide your mail into smaller portions.

Diarrhoea and/or constipation can be complicated for certain cancers like colon cancer pancreatic cancer and lymphoma. Some cancer treatments such as chemotherapy and radiation might also cause these issues. Talk to your doctor in address this problem.

Flu viruses mainly lead to nausea and diarrhoea which can rapidly cause loss of water and electrolytes. You can have ice chips are salted broth (it's a good option if you can tolerate it well). You might also go for sugar free sports drink but be aware that some of them have colouring and artificial sweeteners. Choose the purest one and keep a few bottles always beside you.

- **Homemade electrolyte drink**

Beth Zupec-Kania, consultant nutritionist has suggested this home remedy for electrolyte replacement.
1. ½ teaspoon Morton lite salt
2. ½ teaspoon baking soda
3. 4 cups water

Dissolve salt and baking soda in water. Drink 1 cup every two hours. Test your blood sugar level regularly. If it is below 55 mg/dL, sip 1 to 2 tablespoons of apple juice. When you are able to eat again, start with small meals of bland foods. Add small amounts of mayonnaise, butter, or coconut oil. Good food choices include avocado, soups, or keto shakes (almond or coconut milk, cream, vanilla, stevia).

- **Emergency care**

Have your personal medical information Handy. You can keep it on your mobile phone and present it to consultant or in case of any emergency. Struggling to access your record is only a waste of time which can lead you to danger in emergency cases. If your treatment team offers and excess to upload your medical records timely, just do it! Make sure that you are able to access the portal from your Smartphone, so that your records are only e a click away from you. If you keep your records in pen and paper form mixture to keep it together in a zip-lock bag for easy access at the time of need. Keep a summary of the following points always with you:

• Details of your ketogenic diet plan

• Normal-for-you blood glucose and ketone measurements

• Normal-for-you sodium levels (especially if levels are on the low end)

- Your health care team's contact information, including names, phone, fax, and email.

- **Vacations**

Make some time to live your life to the fullest by going on vacation despite your cancer treatment. Mini vacations are easier it won't burden your diet and your treatment. Take advantage of your skin dual treatment break to enjoy a special time with family and friends. Before going in on to vacations you have to do some homework like- learning what keto friendly foods are available at your destination! Travel takes you to different food custom and language; you will be staying in hotel where you might not get what you had thought of eating as your meal. So always be aware of what keto foods are available in hotels on which you can feed without being worried about carbs.

LONG TERM REWARDS OF KETOGENIC DIET:

If you have been following a low-carb ketogenic plan for several years, now you are absolutely keto-adapted. It is no longer a diet; it's a way of life for you, and a satisfying one! It has many lifelong benefits as mentioned below:

- weight loss (if this is a goal)
- improved blood pressure
- improved metabolic health
- improved insulin sensitivity
- lower levels of inflammation
- more consistent energy and better endurance
- less reliance on scheduled meal times
- improved mitochondrial health
- a sharper mind
- an amazing quality of life
- the potential for a longer lifespan
- the knowledge needed to make better food choices
- all the other benefits that come with understanding

the role that nutrition plays in health and disease

NOTES:

In this chapter you have learn about the physical and mental tips to lead an anticancer life. If you keep track and follow all the steps correctly you will live a happy life while dealing with cancer. If you are dealing with cancer your life doesn't end there! There is still a ray of hope which lies within you; you just have to find out the way you need to lead your life to fight from cancer.

REFERENCE:

CONCLUSION

When I hear something new it makes me curious in a philosophical and scientific way. I do research on it and note down everything I like. The main purpose of writing this book is to pass on the knowledge that I gained about cancer and ketogenic diet to help people to lead a healthy life while fighting cancer. I want you to help up in every possible way regarding your daily life style which can prevent you from suffering from cancer.

Everything happens in our body according to the food we consume and the air we inhale! So why not keep your food healthy? We cannot control the air we breathe but we have full control over our diet. Today food is loaded with lot of junks which is carbohydrate! Yes carbohydrate is a junk. Do it is a fuel for energy in our body system, it is also the reason of many e diseases. It is not necessary that we can only live on carbohydrates. Life is surely possible if you restrict your carbohydrate intake. If we didn't have a backup system of fuel source in our body human existence would have not been possible since ages. Body reacts to carbohydrate restriction in similar way as it reacts while fasting or starvation: by flipping a metabolic swap which allows store fat to be used as fuel.

When all is said and done, the ketogenic diet is simply a different mix of familiar foods, and ultimately you are the one who gets to decide what you eat. Where that takes you is an unknown. We are on a journey of discovery, and like the early explorers, we will uncover new worlds as we keep putting one foot in front of the other.

KETO RECIPES

Want right weight forever? Follow the recipes....

➤ Meat recipe

1. Corned Beef & Cabbage

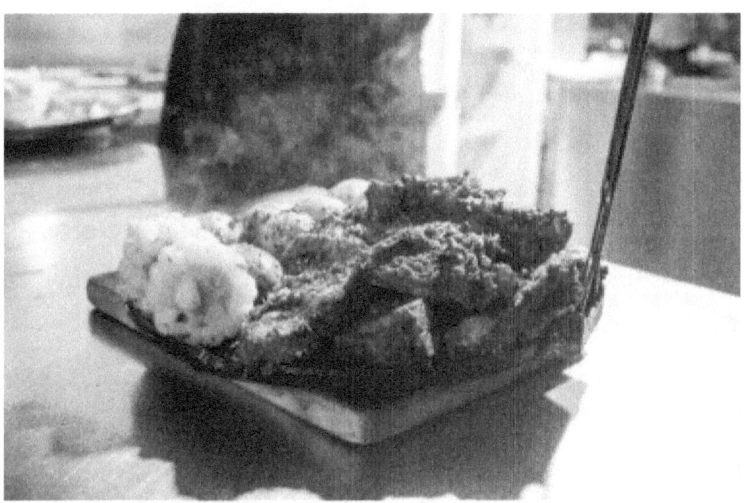

Serves: 6
Ingredients
- 5 medium carrots
- 1 head cabbage
- 1½ lbs. red potatoes
- ½ teaspoon whole allspice berries
- 1 teaspoon dried thyme
- 3 whole black peppercorns
- 3 peeled and smashed garlic cloves
- 2 small bay whole leaves
- 1 small onion, peeled and cut in quarter
- 4 cups water
- 3-4 lbs. corned beef brisket

DIRECTIONS

1. Put corned beef, thyme, all spice, peppercorns, garlic cloves, onion quarters and water in an Instant Pot, then lock the lid.

2. Set the cooker to Manual for 90 minutes and then cook.

3. Once the time elapses, switch off the Instant Pot and let the pressure release naturally in about 10 minutes.

4. Take out the meat from the liquid and set onto a plate. Cover the meat using a tin foil, and let it cool for around 15 minutes. Meanwhile, prepare the veggies.

5. Once ready, add in cabbage, carrot and potato to the liquid in the pressure cooker and secure the lid. Set it to manual and cook for around 10 minutes.

6. Quickly release the pressure. Now carefully open the lid. Remove the veggies using a slotted spoon.

7. Serve the veggies with corned beef. You can moisten the veggies and meat with the cooking liquid.

Nutritional Information per Serving: Calories: 318, Fat: 15.8g, Carbs: 1.6g, Protein: 39.4g

2. Lamb Curry

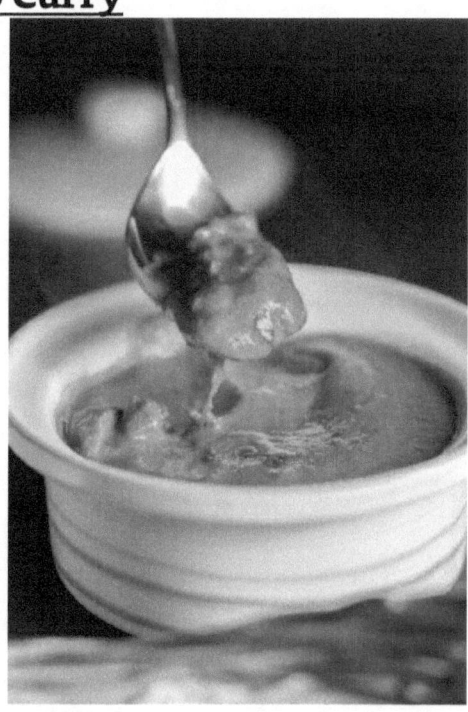

Serves: 6

Ingredients
- 3 medium carrots, sliced
- 1 medium diced zucchini
- 1 medium diced onion
- 1 (14 ounce) can tomatoes
- 1 tablespoon ghee
- Pinch of black pepper + to taste
- 1 ½ tablespoons yellow curry powder
- ¼ teaspoon sea salt + to taste
- ½ cup coconut milk
- Cilantro, chopped (optional)
- Juice of ½ lemon
- fresh ginger, 1-inch piece, grated
- 1 ½ lbs. cubed lamb stew meat
- 4 cloves garlic, minced
- ¾ teaspoon turmeric, optional

DIRECTIONS

1. Mix coconut milk, meat, grated ginger, minced garlic, pepper, salt and lime juice in a container and marinate the meat for about 30-60 minutes.

2. Once ready, mix the marinated meat with ghee, tomatoes and their juice, curry powder, carrots and onions in an instant pot.

3. Lock and secure the lid then set to Manual. Cook on high for about 20 minutes.

4. After 20 minutes, let the Instant Pot sit for around 15 min to release the pressure naturally. Discharge the residual steam by flipping the steam release handle to 'Venting'.

5. Open the lid and then set the Instant Pot to sauté. Then add in diced zucchini and simmer the mixture for 5-6 minutes or until the sauce is slightly thickened and the zucchini is tender.

6. Serve the lamb curry with cauliflower rice garnished with chopped cilantro.

Nutritional Information per Serving: Calories: 230, Fat: 9g, Carbs: 11g, Protein: 25g

3. Instant Pot Pork and Kraut

Serves: 4

Ingredients
- 1 cup filtered water
- 3 cloves garlic peeled & sliced
- 2 large onions sliced or chopped
- 2-3 lbs. pork roast
- 2 tablespoons organic coconut oil or ghee Freshly Ground Black Pepper
- Sea salt
- 4-6 cups sauerkraut, divide
- Optional
- 1 lb. hot dogs nitrate free, grass fed beef
- ½ lb. kielbasa nitrate free, grass fed beef

DIRECTIONS

1. Season the pork shoulder with pepper and salt and then set aside.

2. Brown the pork roast in a large skillet with coconut oil then brown it on all sides over high heat, including on the edges.

3. Put the browned pork roast in the cooking pot of your instant pot. Add garlic, water, onions and add additional salt and pepper as per your taste.

4. Cook the meat on Meat/Stew function for approximately 35 minutes.

5. Naturally release pressure and then add in half of the sauerkraut and save the rest to be eaten raw to help preserve beneficial bacteria (probiotics).

6. Cook the mixture at high pressure for about 5 minutes to flavor the meat. In case the meat is tough, you may need to cook it for 15 minutes!

7. Quick release the pressure and then add in kielbasa and hot dogs if using.

8. Cook for about 5 minutes at high pressure but not for longer as this might break the hot dogs apart.

9. Quick release pressure and then allow the food to rest for a few minutes. Serve with raw sauerkraut and enjoy.

Nutritional Information per Serving: Calories 295.6, Fat 4.3g, Carbs 17.9g, Protein 6.0g

4. **Turkey and Gravy**

Serves: 6

Ingredients
- 2 bay leaf
- Half cup dry white wine
- 1 cups bone broth
- 2 teaspoons dried sage
- 1 celery rib, diced
- 1 garlic clove, peeled and smashed
- 1 large carrot, diced
- 2 tablespoons coconut oil or ghee
- 1 diced onion, medium size
- Black pepper
- 1 4-5 lb. bone-in, skin-on turkey breast
- Salt to taste
- 1 tablespoon tapioca starch, optional

DIRECTIONS

1. Pat-dry the meat and season with pepper and salt. Press the sauté function on the instant pot; add in the ghee to melt.

2. Once melted, add in the turkey breast to brown with the skin side down for about 5 minutes. Transfer to a plate, but leave the melted fat in the cooking pot.

3. Add in celery root, carrot and onion to the pot and cook on sauté function. Cook for around 5 minutes then stir in sage and garlic. Cook for about 30 seconds, until fragrant.

4. at this point, pour in the wine and cook for around 3-4 minutes, or until it is slightly reduced.

5. Add bay leaf and broth and scrape up browned bits stuck onto the pot's bottom using a wooden spoon.

6. Put the turkey skin side up into the Instant Pot along with accumulated juices. Lock and secure the lid in place and cook for 35 minutes at high pressure.

7. Once done, quick release the pressure and gently open the lid. Put the turkey breast onto a plate or carving board.

8. Cover it loosely with foil, and let it cool down as you make the gravy.

9. To prepare the gravy, transfer the veggies and the cooking liquid into a food processor until smooth.

10. Transfer the gravy to the pot and let it cook until thickened. Once reduced to around 2 cups turn off the cooker and add seasonings.

11. In case you like thick gravy, mix a tablespoon of tapioca starch with a tablespoon of warm water and whisk into the gravy.

12. To serve the turkey breast, slice and top with the hot gravy.

Nutritional Information per Serving: Calories: 330, Carbs: 3.7g, Fat 17.9g, Protein: 38g

➤ SEAFOOD RECIPE

1. <u>10-Minute Instant Pot Salmon</u>

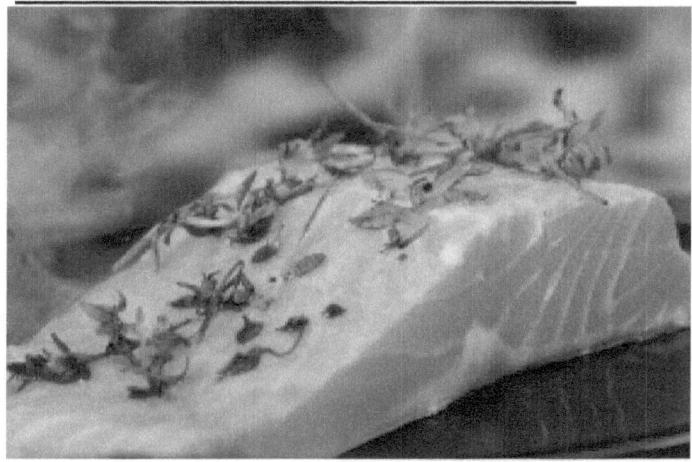

Serves: 4
Ingredients
- 1 tablespoon butter, unsalted
- 1/4 teaspoon black pepper, ground
- 4 fillet salmon
- 1/4 teaspoon salt
- 3 medium lemon
- 1 bunch dill weed, fresh
- 3/4 cup water

DIRECTIONS

1. Put the water and juiced lemon in the bottom of the instant pot then insert the steamer insert.

2. Put the salmon fillets on the steamer insert then sprinkle some fresh dill on top of your salmon fillets and then put a fresh lemon on each of the fillets.

3. Secure the lid in the place set the manual timer to 5 minutes then let cook.

4. As soon as the timer beeps, quick release the steam and then carefully open the lid.

5. Serve the fish with lemon, extra dill and butter. You can also serve with cauliflower rice.

Nutritional Information per Serving: Calories 382, Fat 15g, Carb 4.3g, Protein 41g

2. Steamed Shrimp and Asparagus

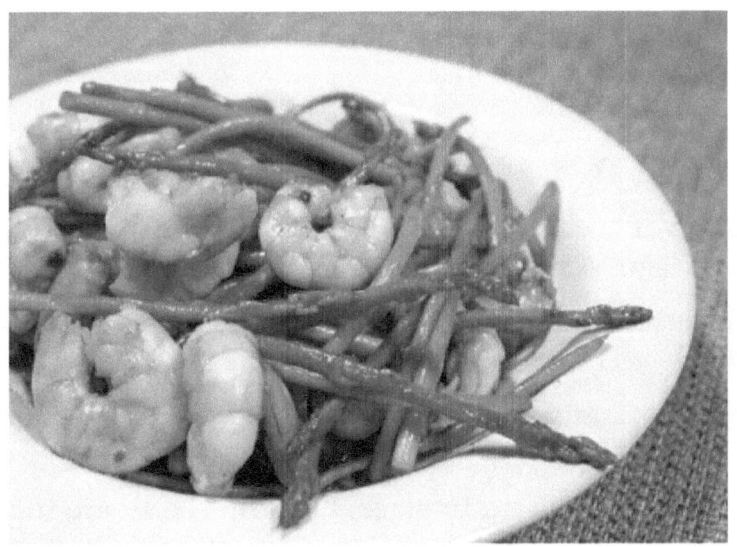

Serves 4

Ingredients
- 1 pound shrimp, frozen or fresh
- ½ tablespoon Cajun seasoning
- 1 bunch of asparagus
- 1 teaspoon olive oil

DIRECTIONS

1. Add a cup of water to the cooking pot of an instant pot. Then insert the steam rack at the bottom.

2. Put the asparagus in a single layer to be the bed for the shell fish. Now place the shrimp on the asparagus.

3. Drizzle with some oil and season with preferred add-ons such as Cajun seasoning.

4. Cover and lock the lid in place. Press on the steam function and set the timer to 2 minutes. If you use fresh shrimp, reduce the time to a minute.

5. Set the pressure to low and set the top knob to sealing. Cook until the instant pot beeps at the end of the cooking.

6. Now move the knob to venting to manually release pressure. Wait until all the pressure has been lost then serve the dish.

Nutritional Information per Serving: Calories 134, Fat 2.71g, Carbs 1.92g, Protein 23.94g

➤ BREAKFAST

The first meal of the day is breakfast so why not to start your day with healthy and tasty keto food. Breakfast should be healthy and packed with energy to start to your day. It should keep you filled until lunchtime, and should definitely pleases your taste buds. It should have a shorter cooking time than preparing meals.

1. Sausage-Broccoli Breakfast

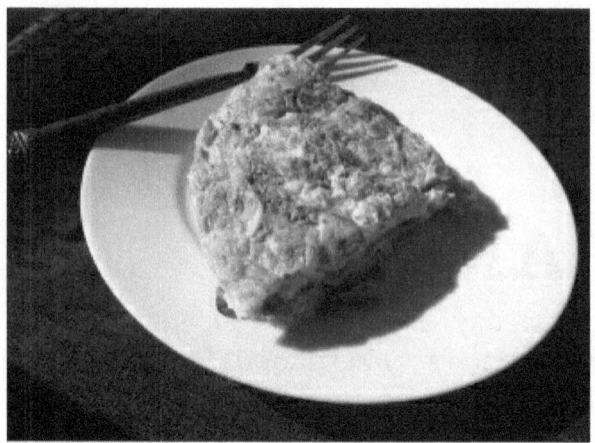

Ingredients: [serves 6-8]

- 1 medium-sized head of broccoli, chopped
- 1 cup cheddar cheese
- 1 lb. breakfast sausage, cooked and sliced
- ¾ cup heavy whipping cream
- 10 eggs
- 2 minced cloves garlic
- Half tsp. black pepper
- ½ tsp. salt or as per your taste

Preparation:

1. Grease the inside of a large slow cooker.
2. Put half the broccoli into the crock-pot. Top it with half the sausage, then half the cheese. Repeat the layer, ending with the cheese.
3. Take another bowl and mix together all the other ingredients until they're well mixed. Pour this mix on the layers in the crock-pot.
4. Cook on low heat for 4-5 hours. The edges should be slightly browned and the centre pretty firm.

Nutritional Info per Serving

- Calories 484
- Dietary Fiber 1.2 g
- Protein 27 g

- Total Carbs 5.5 g
- Total Fat 39 g

2. Florentine Brunch Bake

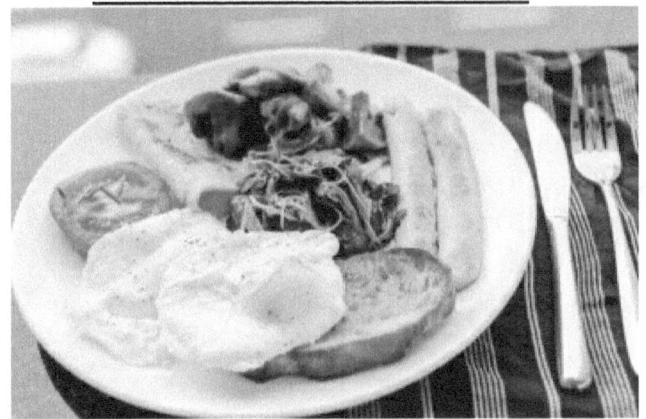

Ingredients: [serves 4-6]

- 1 ½ cups cheddar cheese, grated
- 1 cup of white bread cubes
- 1 8-oz. frozen spinach (packed)
- ½ cup green onion, sliced
- 1 cup sliced, fresh mushrooms
- 6 eggs
- 4-oz heavy cream
- 12-oz milk
- 1.5 tsp. garlic powder
- 1 tsp. Salt (as per taste)
- 1 tsp. black pepper

Preparation:

1. Lightly grease the inner portion of the slow cooker.
2. Layer in the bottom of the crock: a ½ cup of the cheese, half the spinach, half the bread cubes, half the mushrooms, and half the green onions.

3. Repeat the layers.
4. In another bowl, mix the all other ingredients, whisking well. Transfer over the layers in the slow cooker. Do not mix or stir! Sprinkle the remaining half-cup of cheese on the top.
5. Let it cook on high heat for 1 ½-2 hours.

Nutritional Info Per Serving
- Calories 303
- Dietary Fiber 1.7 g
- Protein 20 g
- Total Carbs 12.4 g
- Total Fat 19.6 g

3. Breakfast Pie

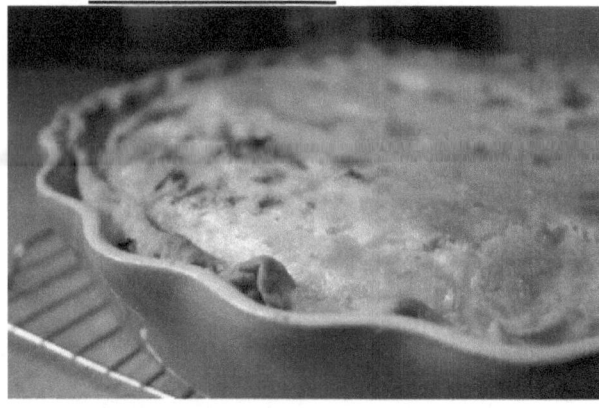

Ingredients: [serves 4-6]
1. 8 eggs, beaten
2. 1 yellow onion, diced
3. salt and pepper
4. 1 sweet potato or yam peeled and shredded
5. 2 tsp. crushed dried basil
6. 1 T. garlic powder
7. 1 lb. pork sausage, crumbled

Preparation:

1. Generously grease the slow cooker with coconut oil.

2. Put your shredded sweet potato in the crock, and then all the other ingredients. Combine it by stirring.

3. Cover and cook on low for 6-8 hours.

NUTRITIONAL INFO PER SERVING
- Calories 379
- Dietary Fiber 1.4 g
- Protein 23 g
- Total Carbs 9.4 g
- Total Fat 27.3 g

DESSERT

1. Blueberry Fat Bombs

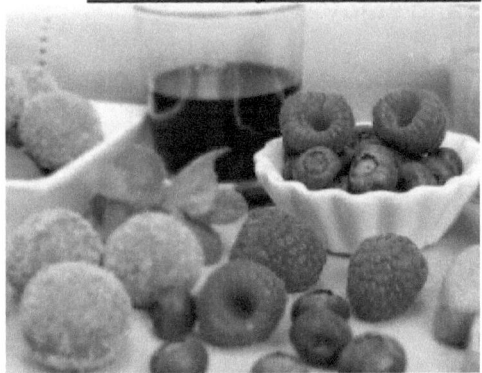

Preparation time: 6-10 min

Cooking time: 3-5 min

Serve: 24

Ingredients:

- 1 stick butter
- 1 cup blueberries
- Half cup softened cream cheese
- 6-oz coconut oil
- Sugar-free sweetener to taste
- ¼ cup coconut cream

Directions:

1. Place the butter and coconut oil in a saucepan and let it melt over low flame. Put down the flame set the saucepan aside.

2. Meanwhile, combine the coconut cream, softened cream cheese and berries in a food processor and pulse until it becomes smooth.

3. Add the melted butter and coconut oil and blend for 15-20 seconds until combined and smooth.

4. Taste and add sugar-free sweetener to your taste. Pour the mixture into molds and freeze for 1-2 hours until they have hardened.

5. Remove from the molds and enjoy.

Nutrition Facts (per serving)

Total Carbohydrates: 19g

Dietary Fiber: 17g

Net Cabs: 2.5g

Protein: 42g

Total Fat: 14g

Calories: 120

2. Almond Fat Bombs

Preparation time: 5-10 min

Cooking time: 0 min

Serves: 4

Ingredients:

- 60 drops (3/8 tsp.) liquid Stevia
- ¾ cup melted coconut oil
- ½ cup almond butter
- 8 tablespoons (1 stick) salted butter, melted
- 3 tablespoons cocoa

Directions:

1. Put the coconut oil and butter in a saucepan and let it melt over low heat. Add the almond butter, stevia, cocoa and stir well to combine.

2. Place a silicone mold on a small cookie sheet. Pour about 2 tablespoons of mixture into each of silicone candy molds and place in the freezer for an hour.

3. Once hardened, remove from the molds and serve.

4. Keep the leftovers stored in the freezer.

Nutrition Facts (per serving)

Total Carbohydrates: 2g

Dietary Fiber: 0g

Net Cabs: 2g

Protein: 2g

Total Fat: 14 g

Calories: 141

3. Dark & Decadent Chocolate Cake

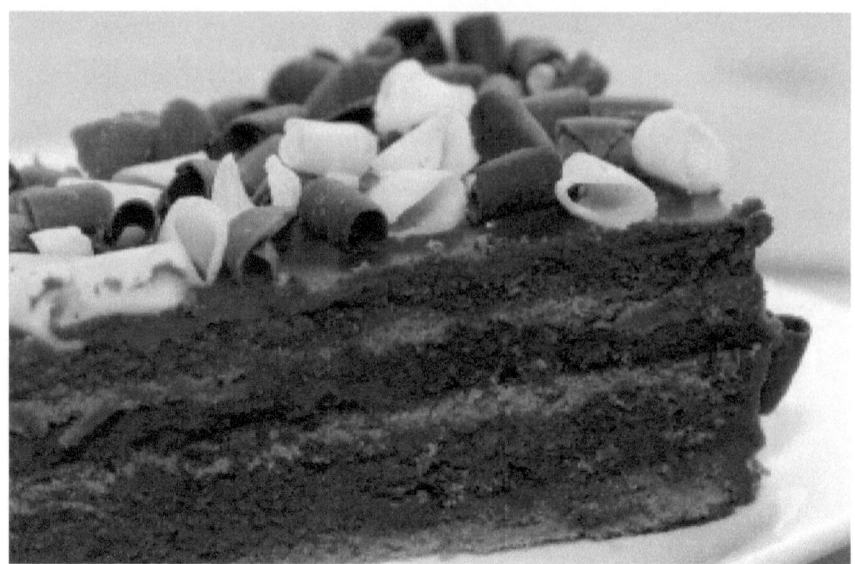

Ingredients: [serves 10]

- 12-oz almond flour
- 2-oz cup whey protein powder (unflavoured)
- 2/3 cup dark cocoa powder
- ¾ cup sugar substitute
- ¼ tsp. Salt to taste
- 2 tsp. baking powder
- ¾ cup unsweetened coconut milk
- ½ cup sugar-free chocolate chips
- 1 tsp. vanilla extract
- ½ cup butter, melted

Preparation:

1. Grease the crock of a large slow cooker with coconut oil.
2. In another bowl, mix together all the dry ingredients (almond flour, sweetener, baking powder, protein powder, cocoa powder, and salt).

3. In the butter add eggs, coconut milk, and vanilla extract. Stir to mix well.
4. Stir in the chocolate chips, distributing them evenly throughout the batter.
5. Pour into the slow cooker. Cook on low for 2 ½ -3 hours. It should still be like a 'pudding cake' at about 2 ½ hours and more firm by the 3-hour mark, so choose your desired consistency.
6. Turn off the slow cooker and allow the cake to cool with the cover off for about 25 minutes.
7. Cut and serve.

Nutritional Info per Serving

Calories 275

Dietary Fiber 5.4 g

Protein 9.9 g

Total Carbs 11.6 g

Total Fat 22.9 g

4. Believe-It-Or-Not Low Carb Cheesecake

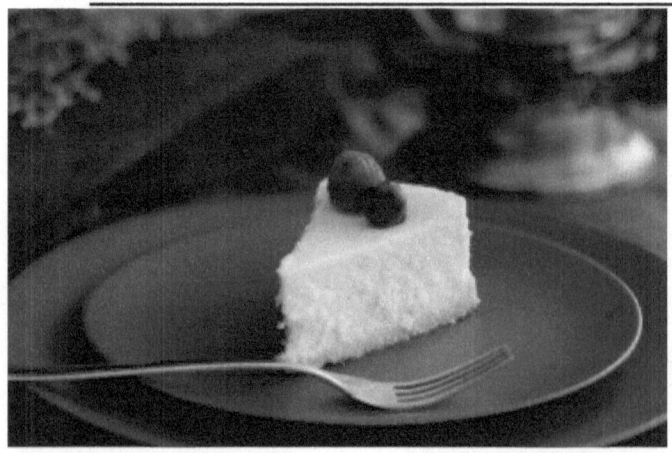

Ingredients: [serves 8]

For the crust:

- 2 ½ T. butter, melted
- ¾ cup graham cracker crumbs
- 1 tsp. Truvia sweetener (1 packet)
- ¼ tsp. salt
- ¼ tsp. cinnamon

For the filling:

- 4 T. plus 2 tsp. Truvia sweetener (16 packets)
- 1 T. flour
- 12 oz. cream cheese, room temperature
- 1 tsp. vanilla extract
- 2 eggs
- 1 cup sour cream

Preparation:

1. Mix the crust ingredients together and press them into the bottom and 1-inch up the sides of a 6-inch spring-form pan. Pack it firmly.
2. Use a standing mixer to combine the very soft cream cheese, the flour, the remaining Truvia, and the salt. Beat about 2 minutes at medium speed until it becomes smooth.
3. Add the eggs and the vanilla-extract and blend well, scraping down the sides of the bowl.
4. Add the sour cream and blend well. Pour the mixture into the spring-form pan.
5. Put a rack in the bottom of your slow cooker. Then add enough water in the bottom to have about a half-inch. Set the filled spring-form pan on the rack.
6. Put a triple layer of paper towel over the top of the crock-pot and put the lid on top of them.

7. Put the slow cooker on high and cook for 120 minutes. Do not lift the lid!
8. Turn off the slow cooker and let it stand undisturbed until it's cooled, about an hour.
9. Remove the lid and the paper towels. Gently lift out the spring-form pan and set it on a cooling rack for about an hour until it comes to room temperature.
10. Cover the cheesecake (in the pan still) with plastic wrap and refrigerate overnight.
11. Remove the cheesecake from the pan. Undo the spring closure on the side of the pan and lift it up and away.
12. Slice, serve, and savor!

Nutritional Info PerServing

Calories 292

Dietary Fiber< 1 g

Protein 6 g

Total Carbs 11.7 g

Total Fat 26.3 g

➤ VEGGIES RECIPES

1. Sweet and Orangey Brussels Sprouts

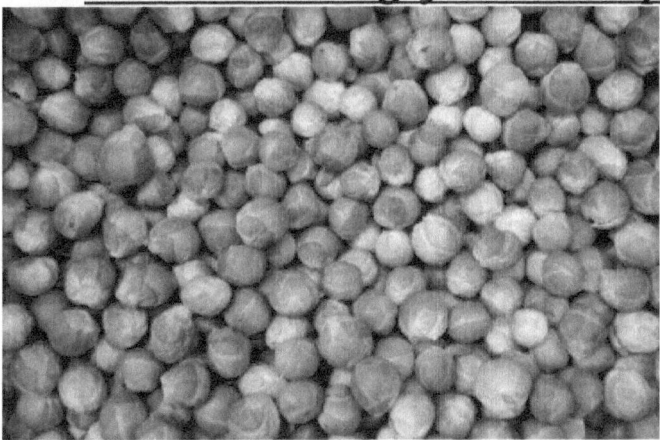

Serves 8

Ingredients

- ½ tsp salt to taste
- 1 tsp grated orange zest
- 1/4 tsp black pepper to taste
- 1 tbsp Earth Balance buttery spread
- 2 tbsp maple syrup
- 2 pounds Brussels sprouts (1.5 pounds when trimmed)
- 1/4 cup orange juice

Directions

1. Trim Brussels sprouts and rinse under cold water.

2. Add all ingredients into the instant pot then cover it. Make sure that the quick release switch is closed.

3. Next, set the time to 3-4 minutes if the sprouts are whole and of good size and 2-3 minutes if the sprouts are small and cut into half. You can reduce the time if you like them harder.

4. When the time lapses, press the off button then proceed to release pressure using the quick release method.

5. Stir well until the sauce covers the Brussels sprouts then serve.

Nutritional Information per Serving: Calories 65, 2g Fat, Protein 3g, Carbs 12g

2. Spiced Potato and Cauliflower

Serves: 4-6

Ingredients

- 1 teaspoon Roasted Cumin Powder
- 1/2 tsp Garam Masala
- 1-2 tsp Coriander Powder
- 1/2 tsp Turmeric Powder
- 1/4-1/2 teaspoon cayenne
- 1 tsp salt
- 1 tsp finely chopped ginger

- 1 medium chopped tomato
- 1 cup Yukon gold potatoes, sliced
- 2 cups cauliflower florets
- 2 tablespoons chopped cilantro
- 2-4 green chillies or 2 jalapeños
- 1 teaspoon cumin seeds
- 1/2 cup onion, sliced
- 1 tablespoon ghee or olive oil

Directions

1. Add cumin seeds in an instant pot then press on the sauté function and allow them to sizzle.

2. Then add the red potatoes, green chilles and onions. Cook these ingredients for a minute or so.

3. Then add in chopped garlic and sauté for about 1 minute more. Add in salt and chopped tomatoes and sauté for 2 more minutes.

4. Now add in cauliflower florets and stir gently. Cancel the sauté function and set the instant pot to manual.

5. Cook the dish for up to a minute based on the size of potatoes and the cauliflower florets.

6. Open the lid and naturally release pressure. In case you find any liquid at the bottom, sauté for a few more minutes.

7. Garnish the meal with cilantro if you like.

Nutritional Information per Serving: Calories 123, Fat 10.9g, Carbs 4.4g, Protein 1.5g

3. Stir-Fried Broccoli

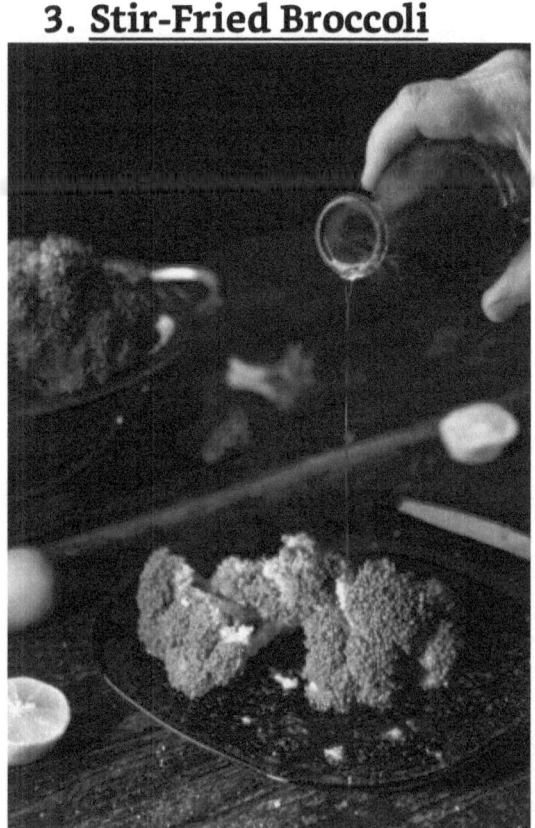

Serves 4

Ingredients

- 6 tablespoons chicken or vegetable stock
- 1 slice of ginger, fresh and peeled
- 1 bunch of broccoli stems cut into flowerets
- 1 large, crushed and peeled garlic clove
- 2 tablespoons Keto friendly sauce
- 2 tablespoons olive oil
- Salt

Directions

1. In the Instant Pot, heat oil until it's very hot. Then stir fry ginger and garlic to obtain a golden colour.

2. Now stir fry broccoli until bright green, then sprinkle with salt. Transfer the mixture into the steamer basket of your cooker.

3. Then pour the sauce and stock into the bottom of the cooker, and lower the basket in.

4. Close and secure the lid, press manual then set the timer to 2 minutes. Use the quick release method to release pressure after the 2 minutes then remove the steamer basket.

5. Serve it.

Nutritional Information per Serving: Calories 156, Fat 12.4g, Carbs 1.9g, Protein, 6.1g, Fiber 3.9g

4. Butternut Squash Pasta

Serves: 6

Ingredients

- 3 cups fresh spinach, rough chopped
- cups homemade bone broth
- Salt and pepper, to taste
- 1 pound penne pasta (low carb)
- 1 tablespoon bacon grease
- ½ medium butternut squash cut in one inch pieces
- 1 tablespoon butter
- 1 small chopped onion
- 2 chopped cloves of garlic
- 2 tablespoons olive oil
- 6 slices bacon, chopped
- Grated Parmesan cheese, optional

Directions

1. Press Browning or Sauté function on your Instant Pot and

allow to heat.

2. To the cooking pot, add bacon grease and sauté until crisp. Then remove the bacon from cooking pot and drain it. Reserve the cooking grease.

3. Now add in oil along with the onions and sauté until the onions are cooked through.

4. Then add in garlic, sauté for a minute and follow with pepper, salt, butter, pasta, bacon grease, bacon and the squashes.

5. Lock the lid in place and set the timer for 4 minutes. Cook until beep sounds then quick release pressure.

6. Carefully open the lid and mix in spinach to the cooking pot.

7. Serve with cheese if you like.

Nutritional Information per Serving: Calories 151, Fat 12.4g, Carbs 6.2g, Protein 5.4g

➤ SOUPS

1. Keto Instant-Pot Soup Low-Carb

Serves 6

Ingredients

- 1 tablespoon Dijon mustard
- 4 dashes hot pepper sauce
- 6 slices cooked turkey bacon, diced
- 2 cups grated Cheddar cheese
- 1 cup half-and-half
- 1 large yellow onion, diced
- 1 (32 fluid ounce) container chicken stock
- Ground black pepper
- Salt
- 1 chopped green bell pepper
- 1 tablespoon onion powder
- 1 head cauliflower, chopped
- 2 minced garlic cloves
- 1 tbsp olive oil

Directions

1. Sauté garlic and onion in an instant pot. Cook the mixture for around 3 minutes, or until browned.

2. Then add in onion powder, green bell pepper, cauliflower, salt and pepper. Pour in the stock and secure the lid.

3. Press on the soup button and set cook time to 15 minutes. Once done, quick release and wait for 5 minutes.

4. Then unlock the lid and add in hot sauce, Dijon, turkey bacon, half-and-half and cheddar cheese.

5. Press on the sauté function and now cook for around 5 minutes, or until bubbles appear. Serve it.

Nutritional Information per Serving: Calories 347 kcal, Fat 25.6g Carbs: 13.4g, Protein 17.7g

2. <u>Chicken and Wild Rice Soup Recipe</u>

Serves 6

Ingredients

- 1 teaspoon pepper
- 1 teaspoon poultry seasoning
- 1 tablespoon parsley
- 48 ounce chicken broth
- 1 teaspoon salt
- ½ teaspoon Italian seasoning
- 1 teaspoon minced garlic
- ¼ teaspoon rosemary
- 1 box Uncle wild rice
- 1 cup diced celery
- 1 cup diced carrot
- 1 tablespoon olive oil
- 3 chicken breast, diced into cubes
- 1 cup diced onions

Directions

1. Press the sauté button then add a tablespoon of oil, celery, carrots and onions.

2. Cook the ingredients until cooked through, or for around 5 minutes. Then add in 1/3 cup of chicken broth while scrapping the pan.

3. Follow with the diced chicken, seasons, 3 and ½ cups chicken broth and wild rice.

4. Close the lid and set cook time to 6 minutes. Wait for a few minutes for the instant pot to come into pressure.

5. Once cooking is done, natural release for about 7 minutes then quick release. You may need to place a towel on the steam release for soup not to spew out of it.

6. At this point, carefully open the lid and shred the diced chicken chunks using a fork.

7. Press the sauté button and add the chicken stock into the instant pot and sauté until you get your preferred consistency.

8. Let the soup boil for some time then turn off the pressure cooker.

Nutritional Information per Serving: Calories 286, Fat 20g, Carbs 13g, Protein 23g

3. Keto Bacon Cheeseburger Soup

Serves: 6

Ingredients

- 1 cup shredded sharp cheddar cheese
- 6 ounce bacon, chopped
- 4 ounces cream cheese
- 2 large carrots, diced
- 4 cups beef or chicken broth
- Sea salt to taste
- 4 cups cauliflower, chopped
- 2 stalks celery, diced
- 1 large onion, diced
- 1½ pounds hamburger

Directions

1. Press the sauté button on the instant pot and brown the bacon for a few seconds.

2. Brown the ground beef until it is cooked through then remove from the cooking pot.

3. Add the veggies and sauté until soft. You can add in coconut oil if using lean meat.

4. Pour in broth and lock the lid. Cook for 7 minutes and then quick release the steam.

5. At this point, use an immersion blender to make puree of the vegetable inside pot.

6. Then stir in the cheeses and blend to incorporate. Also stir in the hamburger and bacon back in and allow sitting for a few minutes to warm up.

7. Serve and enjoy.

Nutritional Information per Serving: Calories 330, Fat 17g, Protein 21g, Carbs 6g

4. **Curried Cream of Broccoli Soup**

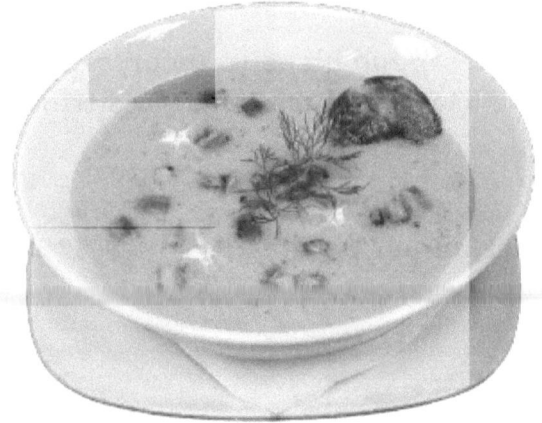

Serves 6

Ingredients

- 1½ pounds broccoli, chopped
- 4 cups bone broth or chicken stock
- Black pepper, freshly-ground
- 1 cup full-fat coconut milk
- ¼ cup peeled apple, diced
- Chives, garnish
- Leftover Kalua Pork, crisped in a pan
- 1 tablespoon Indian curry powder
- Kosher salt

- 2 medium shallots, chopped
- 2 tablespoons olive oil, coconut oil or ghee
- 3 medium leeks, chopped

Directions

1. Prepare and chop the broccoli, leeks or onions. Press the sauté button on Instant Pot, add fat and then cook the shallots, leeks, curry powder and salt.

2. Cook for 5 minutes, stirring occasionally until the curry is fragrant. Now stir in chopped broccoli and apple.

3. Follow with broth and ensure the Instant Pot isn't more than 2/3rd full. Cook the mixture (use manual function to set the cook time) for 5 minutes.

4. Then turn off the cooker and quick release the pressure. Now open the lid and transfer the ingredients into a blender. Puree to produce a green aromatic soup.

5. Add in coconut milk. Season it with salt and some pepper. Continue to blend as desired.

6. You can add crisped-up meat such as Kalua pork and garnish with chives. Save up to 4 days and freeze for a few months.

Nutritional Information per Serving: 125 Calories, Fat 10g, Carbs 18g, Protein 4.0g

RESOURCES

Ketogenic Diets and Cancer: Emerging Evidence. (n.d.), from https://www.ncbi.nlm.nih.gov/pmc/articles/PMC6375425/

Mitochondrial dysfunction in cancer. - PubMed - NCBI. (n.d.). Retrieved from https://www.ncbi.nlm.nih.gov/m/pubmed/26327844/

The books I referred are:

Hoffman, V. (n.d.). Ketogenic Instant Pot Cookbook: The best 100 Keto Instant Pot Recipes To Lose Weight and Being Healthy! - Kindle edition by Virginia Hoffman. Cookbooks, Food & Wine Kindle eBooks @ Amazon.com. Retrieved from https://www.amazon.com/Ketogenic-Instant-Pot-Cookbook-Recipes-ebook/dp/B079SP375M

Hoffman, H. (n.d.). Ketogenic Diet: Rapid Weight Loss Snacks VOLUME 1: Lose Up To 30 Lbs. In 30 Days by Henry Brooke. Retrieved from https://www.goodreads.com/book/show/27134477-ketogenic-diet

Ketogenic Diet: 30 Fast Fat Loss Slow Cooker Recipes (Ketogenic Diet, Ketogenic Recipes, Ketogenic Cookbook, Ketogenic diet for weight loss, diabetes diet, ketogenic) - Kindle edition by Sara Givens. Cookbooks, Food & Wine Kindle eBooks @ Amazon.com. (n.d.). Retrieved from https://www.amazon.com/Ketogenic-Diet-Cookbook-diabetes-ketogenic-ebook/dp/B00Y9F5YB2

Kaplan, J. (n.d.). Ketogenic Diet: James Kaplan: 9781523333974. Retrieved from https://

www.bookdepository.com/Ketogenic-Diet-James-Kaplan/9781523333974

Jane, E. (n.d.). A Year of Fat Bombs: 52 Seasonal Sweet &Savory Recipes (Ketogenic Diet): Elizabeth Jane: 9780995534544: Amazon.com: Books. Retrieved from https://www.amazon.com/Year-Fat-Bombs-Seasonal-Ketogenic/dp/0995534543

Keto for Cancer: Ketogenic Metabolic Therapy as a Targeted Nutritional Strategy: 9781603587013: Medicine & Health Science Books @ Amazon.com. (n.d.). Retrieved from https://www.amazon.com/Keto-Cancer-Ketogenic-Metabolic-Nutritional/dp/1603587012

www.ingramcontent.com/pod-product-compliance
Lightning Source LLC
Chambersburg PA
CBHW030633220526
45463CB00004B/1505